#MADBACK

HOW TO STOP THE HURTING AND RECLAIM YOUR LIFE, EASILY, NOW

The Holistic Research On Back And Neck Pain,
That You Have Been Looking For, Towards
A Pain-Free Back And Neck, and
A Life Full Of Joy, Freedom, Vitality & Sexuality

PATRICK LEE

M.Sc. Researcher
Human Spinal Neuromechanics

Perspectis, Inc.

1 First Canadian Place, Ste. 350

Toronto, ON, Canada M5X 1C1

ISBN: 978-0-9938841-0-8

DEDICATION

This book is dedicated to my parents, family, colleagues, and back sufferers around the world.

CONTENTS

PART THREE
The Secret of Your Back - What Keeps It Happy

PART FOUR
You Are Your Spine

PART FIVE
New Paradigm for a Pain-Free Back, a Strong Spine, and a Vibrant Life

PROLOGUE

Why Are Mad Backs Everywhere?

Is your back mad at the discomfort if feels when you need to work on the computer for a while? *Is your back mad at the sore it gets in the middle of your car ride home from your work? Is your back mad at the pain it feels when you are reading a good book? Is your back mad at the squirm it couldn't stop in the middle of your favorite TV show you want to enjoy? Is your back mad at the seemingly endless visits to doctor offices that still left you in pain? Is your back mad at being told that it has to put up with the discomfort or pain for the rest of your life?*

Has your back been suffering from a pain or discomfort that hinders your joy of life? *Has your back pain or discomfort been holding you back from your favorite outdoor activities? Does you back start to get painful 20-minutes into your car ride? Does your back become stiff or painful after sitting in front of a computer? Does your back discomfort make you squirm in the middle of watching a movie or a TV show?*

Have your back problems been holding you back from going on the vacation that you have longed for? *Have your back issues been holding you back from taking the trip to see your loved ones, such as your parents, your children or your grandchildren?*

Or

- Is your back frustrated at its nagging discomfort, stiffness, fatigue or pain that doesn't seem to stop?

- Is your back mad at the seemingly countless visits to doctors'

1

offices that still left it in pain?

- Is your back mad at the seemingly countless products that claimed to work, but didn't?

- Is your back mad at the lack of exercise and care it deserves and needs?

- Is your back mad at the seemingly authoritative conclusions that it has to put up with the pain for the rest of your life?

- Is your back mad at the possibility that you may outlive it someday?

- Is your back mad at the poor support it gets when sitting at work, at home, at ball games, in cars or on airplanes?

- Is your back mad that it can't keep up with what you want to do in life?

- Is your back mad that it didn't get the care it needed until it was hit by pain?

If your answer is 'yes' to any of these questions, you are not alone. According to the American Association of Orthopedic Surgeons, 1 in 3 American adults are afflicted with back pain each year, which means about 60 – 70-million American adults have had, are having or are going to have back pain within this calendar year alone. Most of these sufferers' backs are frustrated and mad, because after five to six costly trials of different categories of care and remedies, they still have yet to find something that can help them effectively get the pain under control. In the case of chronic back pain sufferers, the situation is even more severe. Their backs are more frustrated and even madder.

The artificial world humanity has created around itself is incompatible to the 195,000 years of evolution of our spine and back. Drugs are not helping. Surgeries are often ineffective and have too many uncertainties and side effects. The first line defense taken by most people against back pain is not working. Most initial advices and treatments are often applied to the wrong conditions at the wrong time. The health care system is not effective in resolving these problems. Medical education and training is not waking up to this dilemma. And health policies are not addressing these issues, either.

According to Noreen M. Clark, PhD, director the Center for Managing Chronic Disease at the University of Michigan, Ann Arbor, there exist "extraordinarily burdensome" prescribing practices for patients with chronic pain. Commenting on the more than 2,000 public comments on the web site that addressed this issue at the Institute of Medicine, she said: "It is extraordinary how many people described themselves as collateral damage in the war against drugs. Patients are paying the price for policies not designed for their benefit."

12 Shocking Facts About Your Back

Back pain is pervasive and costly. Did you know:…

1. Eighty percent of Americans will have at least one acute episode of back pain in their life.
2. One in every three American adults is afflicted with back pain each year.
3. Most back pain sufferers are dissatisfied with the first care chosen.
4. Most back pain sufferers are frustrated and mad about the poor effectiveness of the solutions they have tried.
5. Many things people do for their back pain are detrimental to their conditions.
6. Most back pains are caused by trivial movements and are mechanical in nature.
7. Most conventional medical doctors lack training in musculoskeletal health and don't feel confident in treating musculoskeletal conditions.
8. Most back pain sufferers use their family doctor as their first line of defense for back pain.
9. Your back is far more critical to you than your teeth.
10. Yet you are more likely to care for your teeth than you do for your back.
11. Back pain holds you back from many of your dreams.
12. Most back pain can be effectively controlled, without drugs or surgery.

Give your back the care it deserves, now. Turn your mad back into a happy back today.

9 Secret Reasons Why Your Back Can Have Its Peace

Keep your head up! Here is the good news:

1. Most likely, the right solution for your back is out there and it can work for you right now.
2. Most back pain can be cut at least in half, by receiving the right care.
3. Most back pain can be prevented or, at least, cut in half by maintaining the right body mechanics -- that is, using the body the right way.
4. Most back pain can be prevented or, at least, cut in half by adopting the right work and lifestyles.
5. Most back pain can be prevented or, at least, cut in half by doing the right exercises regularly.
6. Most back pain can be prevented or, at least, cut in half by using the right aids and tools.
7. Most back pain can be prevented or, at least, cut in half if your spine has received the same level of attention and care that your teeth have.
8. Most back pain can be virtually eliminated if you adopt all the above advice properly.
9. You don't need to put up with back pain for the rest of your life.

This book empowers you to take action to eliminate, prevent or, at least, cut back pain in half by providing practical knowledge, advice and a roadmap to stop the hurting and reclaim your vibrant life.

5 Easy Ways to Make This Book Work For You Fast

This book covers a lot of material. However, if you want to quickly find the right information to help you when your back is mad or when you are pressed for time, simply follow the following 5 Easy Ways to Make this Book Work for You Fast:

1. Go to **PART TWO** if you are in pain and are looking for the right care or the effective solutions to your back problems. This chapter is about how to make your back happy again.
2. Go to **PART THREE** if you want to maintain your spinal

health, or prevent back pain from happening or recurring, or slow down spinal degeneration. This chapter is about how to keep your back happy forever.

3. Go to **PART ONE** if you would like to learn some fundamental secrets about the back and spine that are critical to your understanding of the solutions suitable to help you resolve or prevent your back problem. This chapter is about what makes your back mad.

4. Go to **PART FOUR** if you ever wonder why you should take care of your back, or if you still have any doubt about the importance of taking care of your back and spine. This chapter is about why you are your spine.

5. Go to the **Contents** page and browse through the highlighted materials by your interest.

Although one day, you'll want to read this book completely from cover to cover, by carefully going through the right chapters, you'll save countless hours trying out treatments or products that may not work for you, may delay your recovery, and may even cause you to lose the window of opportunity for a speedy recovery of your back problem. You will also save a mountain of money in eliminating ineffective treatments and products for your condition. You'll also save your body a ton of unnecessary suffering by getting the right care and treatment directly.

One of the secrets to taking care of your back is to learn with your heart, instead of merely understanding knowledge with your mind. You may only begin to take advantage of this knowledge in your daily life when you have taken the information in this book into your heart (when your heart, not only your mind, finds it true and useful).

Reason is very simple. Implementation is the key. And implementation can only be half-hearted if the learning is only by the mind instead of by the heart. How many times have you learned and understood something that you felt made good sense, and you wanted to apply it in your life, but only ended up forgetting it? Only when you can take advantage of knowledge subconsciously, then you can you remember that information when needed.

How do you know you have taken the information to your heart? You know it when you share it with others, naturally. Teaching is learning. Sharing is learning too. This learning is about gaining new insight to the materials you have read and understood, and is about being able to use them naturally. By sharing this new knowledge with your loved ones, your friends, your fellow back health enthusiasts, and your fellow back problem sufferers, you will help your transition from understanding to trusting, and to being confident of taking advantage of these materials for your own back health. How do you make sure that you are able "to share naturally?" There is only one way, begin to share what you learn in this book immediately and frequently with those around you. By doing so, you may even discover deeper truth that this book has yet to cover.

You will be glad that you shared this knowledge, not only because you will benefit from applying these materials for your own good, but also because you will be helping your loved ones, friends, and fellow back health enthusiasts. You will not only be thanked by your back, but also by others backs. By sharing this secret with others, all of you will contribute to a healthier and happier world. All those you share this knowledge with will reap even more rewards in helping the world. What goes around comes around. In this case, it is the health and happiness for you and the world.

Use this book wisely. Get better quickly. Stay healthier easily.

Why I Wrote This Book?

Have you ever wondered why the back and spinal health of an average North American is declining, despite the growing number of books and articles published on this topic and the medical advances that have been made for the treatment of back problems?

The reason is simple: some basic truths have been ignored, for too long.

Most literature unfortunately has been written from the perspective of one single healthcare discipline. For example, most of them have been written from the single perspective of conventional medicine, chiropractic medicine, osteopath medicine, physiotherapy or massage therapy.

A large number of misconceptions still remain untouched. There still exist a significant mismatch between care and conditions. Most patients are still confused about what to do when hit by back pain, and about where to find the suitable care. Most patients are still frustrated with the prolonged, often unnecessary, suffering from back pain. Most patients still don't know what questions to ask when seeing their doctors. Twenty percent of these cases still remain misdiagnosed. Many patients still believe that they have to live with the pain and agony for the rest of their life.

Back pain is a complex issue. No one healthcare discipline has all the answers. It demands and deserves a multidisciplinary view and approach. However, it is also straight forward enough for most of us to take control over.

This book is written from a third-party perspective and is care-discipline neutral. It doesn't favor, nor disfavor, any particular back health care discipline. The author believes that any specific discipline of care discussed in this book could be the best, but also the worst, option for a back pain sufferer, depending on her or his specific condition. This book is only intended to help you better objectively understand the landscape of the back and spinal health care solutions. This book is not an average book that recycles standard information in a laundry list format and proclaims that your back pain will be gone after reading it. Being politically correct or academically perfect is also not amongst the intentions of this book. Feelings may be hurt. Arguments may arise.

This book has only one objective – help you stop the hurting and reclaim your life! It has been written to provide you with the practical information and insight that matters. As folk's wisdom says "effective medicines may be bitter to your taste, and effective advice may be hard on your feelings."

Don't read this book, if you want a book that recycles standard information available to all back pain suffers -- that doesn't hurt but it also doesn't help either.

Do read this book if you want to broaden your horizons, if you want to know things that you can't find in other books, if you want to actively take your own initiatives for the wellbeing of your back and spine, if you want to become a true partner of your back and spine, and if you truly want to control your destiny for your back and spine.

To a large extent, turning your back health around requires a paradigm shift. You must be ready for this shift. This is not going to be easy, because it may require you to adapt to new understandings, new views, new approaches, new habits, and new lifestyles. Simply popping pills or putting yourself on an operation table are not parts of the new paradigm.

This book tells you the truth that matters. This book is a tool that you can use. It provides you with effective secrets that you can zero in on and apply immediately for your particular concern or purpose.

As they say, your clothes become 30% cleaner just by throwing them in water. Simply by learning some of the critical, but rarely known secrets about your back and spine, you will come a long way in getting your back, back in shape.

Most of this knowledge is so simple that a sixth grader can easily understand and master it. Yet it is so rarely known that not even most practicing doctors know these secrets. By reading and mastering the content of this book, you will, at the very least, be able to knowledgably discuss your condition with your doctor.

This book has pioneered a holistic research method and approach, to empower you in your management of your back pain and your spinal health.

It will be the greatest reward to the author, if this book could help you:
- Find the right care for your back problem, faster.
- Save you money and time in your fight against back pain.
- Shorten your suffering from back pain.
- Reduce the intensity of your suffering from back pain.
- Find the true cause of your back pain.
- Prevent recurrences of your back problem.
- Prevent back pain from happening, or
- Have a pain-free back, a strong spine, and a vibrant life full of joy, freedom, friendship, love, happiness, energy, vitality and sexuality.

Acknowledgements

This book didn't come into existence without the generous help and support of many people surrounding me and this book.

My gratitude goes to Dr. Don Fitz-Ritson, Mr. Grant Henderson, Ms. Sigrid Feser, Dr. Chris Oswald, Dr. Bob Hoffman, Mr. Tony Tocco, Mr. Jordan Green, Ms. Jane Ellen, Ms. Linda Sue Perry, Ms. Janice Yan and Mr. Celt Stephenson Li for their candid reviews, critiques, suggestions and advice. They have helped make this book easier to read and easier to use.

My gratitude also goes to the over 2,000 licensed back pain

specialists in the United States, Canada, the United Kingdom, the Netherlands, Australia, Norway, and another 20 countries, whom I had the honor to serve and work with.

My gratitude also goes to the hundreds of thousands of back pain sufferers around the world, whom I have had the privilege to help with some of my specialized know-how and solutions.

Last but not least, my gratitude goes to the millions of back pain sufferers whom I have not had a chance to serve, but whose suffering has inspired me to embark on the journey of writing this book in the first place.

Apologies

While being confident that this book provides many back pain sufferers with a lot of fresh and not-so-easy-to-find facts and insights, as well as a fresh holistic perspective in better dealing with their back and spinal health, this author is also acutely aware of the many shortcomings to this edition of the book.

Due to limited time and resources, this book has mainly focused on getting the most urgently needed information out into the world to help people better relieve, combat, and prevent back and spinal problems. As a result, many other aspects of this book have suffered and need urgent improvements.

Just to name a few, the contents of this book could have been more balanced. The topics more comprehensive. The chapters better organized and formatted. The sentences simplified and better styled. The messages easier to follow. The points better explained and more direct. There could have been fewer typos, missing words, and grammatical mistakes. And there could have been more and better pictures and graphic illustrations to help readers better understand the information and messages of this book. And with each revision, more shortcomings have been identified.

This author is determined to, over time, improve on these identified and those yet to be identified shortcomings to better help and serve its readers.

If this book were a sculpture of David, the real work had just been begun on a huge block of raw marble. At this stage, it has only gained its most basic form and posture. You could see its head, torso, arms, and legs. However, the details of the eyes, nose, lips, ears, hands, feet, and the contour of the muscles are still missing, let alone its facial expression and muscular energy.

I could spend more time trying to perfect this book. But I am no Michelangelo and don't think I could "call" David out of the marble. In other words, I need help from other experts and readers like you to make this book as perfect as it should be. So this book is and shall remain a living project and system.

The existing prevalence of back pain in our society today, after countless excellent books and articles have been written on this topic, serves as a proof. That is why I want to make this book a living project and to work with you, the readers, the sufferers, the caring clinicians, the diligent researchers, and the expert critics, to gradually improve, expand, enrich, update, and perfect it. The simple goal of this project is to help the millions of back pain sufferers stop the hurting. This book needs to become an effective tool in the interests of its readers. And it has been created solely in the interests of its readers and its readers alone.

PART ONE
THE SECRET OF YOUR BACK
- WHAT MAKES IT MAD

Read this chapter to learn fundamental facts about the back and spine that are critical to your understanding of suitable solutions to resolve or prevent your back problems, now and in the future.

1

10 Secret Natures of Your Back You Must Understand

The spine is the foundation of your back. The human spine is a wonder. It is one of the most perfect creations in our world, because it has the perfect shape, the perfect structure, and the perfect function.

It supports your upright posture. It keeps your head on your shoulders. It keeps you standing, sitting, walking, running, and lifting. It allows our body to bend, to rotate, to turn, to move, and to dance. It keeps our body under control. It houses and protects our nerves and allows them to branch out to reach and control every part of our body.

In fact, it is the only spine in the animal kingdom that can support an upright body posture for a prolonged period of time. Our spine allows the most sophisticated functions of our bodies in an upright position. With this natural wonder, human beings can run, jump, and completely free up our two hands for sophisticated functions, such as hunting, planting, fishing, cooking, gathering, building, painting, writing, creating tools, technologies -- indeed -- all civilization and all human history ever, all in an upright posture.

If a chimp was given advanced human intelligence but without a human spine, it would surely,, not achieve much, because the superiority of human beings is largely based on the ability to completely free up our arms and hands for sophisticated functions. Without such ability, the advanced evolution of human intelligence would not have been possible.

Besides the spine, your back also consists of the ligaments and muscles surrounding the spine and the pelvis.

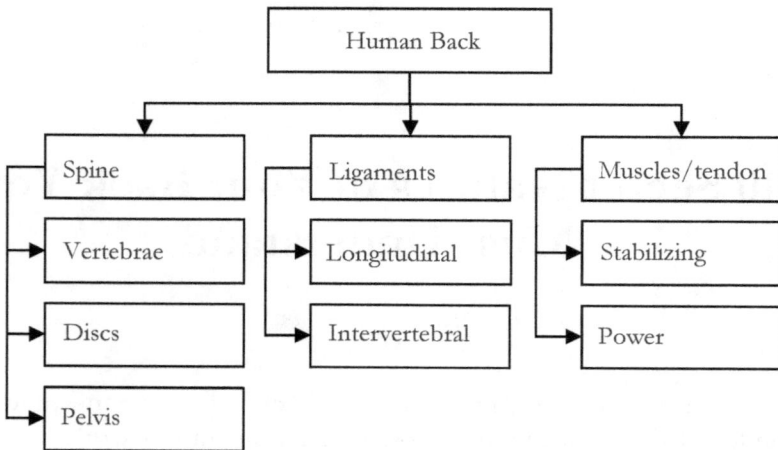

Source: compiled by Patrick Lee.

Fig. 1.1

All of the above mentioned parts of your back, from vertebrae to intervertebral discs, to the ligaments, muscles and tendons around them, and to the pelvis, work as an integrated whole and closely follow a number of natural rules of your body.

There are 10 rarely known but extremely critical secret natures of the back you need to understand. These natures govern the function of your back and body, as well as the sensation and progression of your back pain. To have a strong and pain-free back and spine, you must clearly understand them and take care of your back in the way your body's nature requires.

These 10 secret natures of the back are:

    1.   The interconnected nature of the spine.

2. The self-balancing nature of the body.
3. The loosening nature of the soft tissues
4. The inside-out nature of the body
5. The emotional nature of back pain
6. The vulnerable nature of the spine
7. The self-enforcing nature of poor posture
8. The pervasive nature of spinal degeneration
9. The increase of pain sensors with age
10. And sitting is the new smoking.

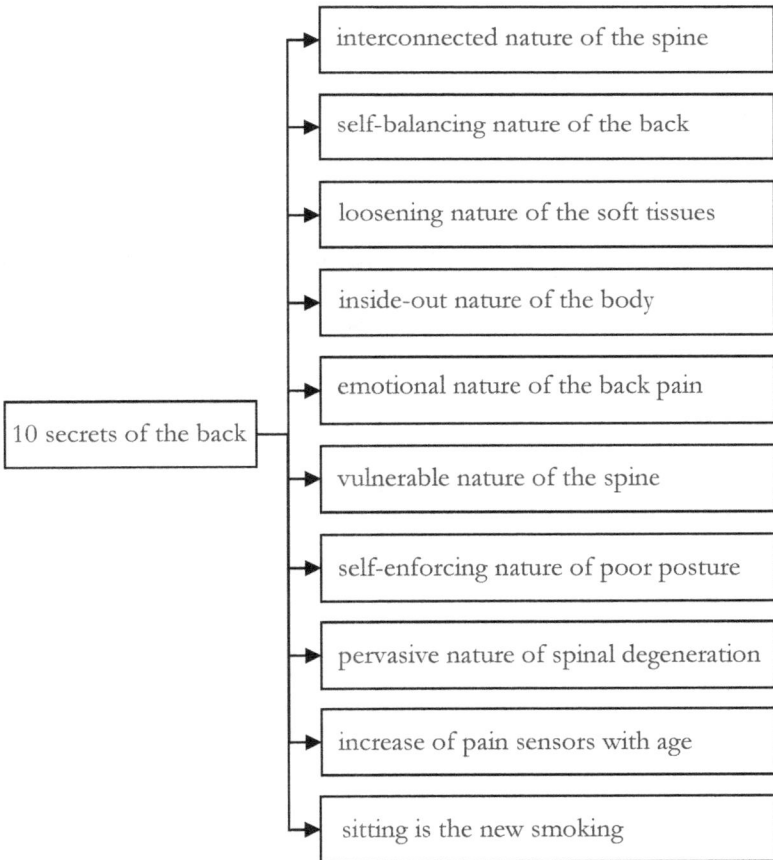

Source: compiled by Patrick Lee
Fig. 1.2

1. The Interconnected Nature of the Spine

Your spine is the core of your back. The health of your back is largely determined by the health of your spine. However, when considering spinal health, we must not only consider the spine itself -- the vertebrae and discs -- but also consider the ligaments and muscles around it.

This is because what hold the back upright are not the spine but the muscles and ligaments surrounding it. Together, the vertebrae, discs, ligaments and muscles form an intricate and interconnected biomechanical system characterized as the tensegrity system.

A tensegrity system is a system that consists of both rigid components for taking compressive forces and flexible components for taking tensile forces. The tensions in each of the rigid or flexible components will affect and determine the tension in all other parts of the same system. The change of tension in each element leads to the change of tension in all other components, rigid and soft.

The term "tensegrity" was coined by American architect Buckminster Fuller, however, the first artistic model of a tensegrity system was created by American sculptor Kenneth Snelson in 1948. On the right is one of the tensegrity models created by Kenneth Snelson. Notice not one of the rigid steel bars is directly connected with each other; however, the entire structure stands solidly from ground up, because the steel bars are pulled up by the flexible steel cables.

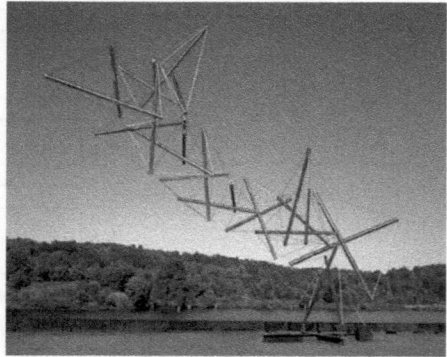

Fig. 1.3 A tensegrity sculpture by contemporary sculptor and photographer, Mr. Kenneth Snelson, image courtesy of Mr. Kenneth Snelson

In the back, the vertebrae are the rigid component responsible for taking on compressive forces, such as body weight, while the muscles are the flexible components responsible for taking on pulling forces, such as those that keep the spine upright. Your spine stands upright because of the pulling of the muscles and ligaments around the vertebrae. Your spine and back will be in trouble if any one of these rigid or flexible components is damaged or malfunctions.

According to the tensegrity principle, the tension and stress in any one vertebrae or muscle will lead to a change in tension in all other vertebrae and muscles in the same system. Never under estimate the damage, malfunction, or imbalance in any one vertebra, disc, ligament, or muscle in your back, because it will cause an imbalance in many other parts of your back. For example, slouching not only affects the vertebrae, discs, ligaments and muscles in the localized lower back, it affects all the other vertebrae, discs, and all the other associated ligaments and muscles.

2. The Self-balancing Nature of the Body

One of the most practical applications of human spinal neuromechanics (an interdisciplinary field that combines neuroscience and biomechanics to study the control of human spinal movement) in back health care is the leverage of our body's self-balancing and coordinating nature, also called it's 'proprioceptive nature.'

Proprioceptive nature is the ability of our body to sense and coordinate the position, motion, and equilibrium. of our body parts automatically and subconsciously. Proprioception is the process in which the proprioceptive nature is in action.

The early concept of proprioception originated as early as the 16th century. In 1557, Julius Caesar Scaliger first described the position-movement sensation as a "sense of locomotion."

In 1826, Charles Bell formulated the idea of a "muscle sense" between the muscles and the brain. His work is considered as one of the first descriptions of physiologic feedback mechanisms.

In 1880, Henry Charlton Bastian suggested the idea of "kinaesthesia" introducing his believe that 'afferent information' (back to the brain) was also coming from other structures besides muscles alone, including tendons, joints, and our skin.

In 1889, Alfred Goldscheider classified kinaesthesia into three types: muscle, tendons, and articular sensitivity.

Then, in 1906, Nobel Prize laureate Charles Scott Sherrington published a landmark work that introduced the term "proprioception" as the awareness of movement derived from muscles, tendons, and joints.

Leveraging proprioceptive nature has wide applications in back health care, such as:

- Improving spinal alignment
- Preventing stiffening backs
- Improving blood circulation to spinal muscles
- Improving hydration to spinal discs
- Maintaining equilibriums
- And maintaining spinal longevity.

When a person sits on a gentle unstable sitting surface, her pelvis will gently rock back and forth like a little boat in a bay with small waves awakened by a gentle summer breeze. Her spine waves like the mast of the boat with the boat. Unlike the fixed mast, the spine immediately starts to balance itself to keep the upper portion of the spine upright while the lower portion bend itself to accommodate the rocking motion of the pelvis, under the subconscious guidance of proprioceptive nature.

In this process the muscles surrounding the spine, especially the deep stabilizing muscles (multifidus, the small muscles directly surrounding the spine) get recruited and activated. Their blood circulation is improved, and their tendency of stiffening and persistent contracting is reduced. At the same time, the hydration process to the spinal discs is activated through a mechanism named imbibition in which the adjacent vertebrae move like a clam opening and closing it shells, and draw fresh body fluid and blood into the spinal discs, and press the old one out, to nurture the discs. The hydration to the spinal discs is therefore improved.

Due to the subconscious balancing action of the spine, slouching is reduced and spinal alignment is improved. Furthermore, the equilibrium and balance function is also activated and utilized.

Static sitting has severe consequences on one's spinal health. In the case of people who spend much of their time sitting at work, at home, or in vehicles and airplanes, the consequences range from:

- The deformed spinal alignment,
- To a static load in the back
- To reduced disc hydration
- To increased peak pressure on spinal discs
- To weakened stabilizing muscles.

With such wide ranging and severe consequences, it is difficult to sustain the benefit of most medical or wellness treatments to the spine or the back. Reducing or even eliminating some or all such consequences will go a long way in helping patients better sustain the benefits of their medical of wellness treatments, hence improving their spinal health.

Leveraging the body's proprioceptive nature is one of the most effective ways to reduce and eliminate some or all such consequences of static sitting.

By stimulating the spine to constantly compensate itself, proprioceptive sitting (sitting on a gentle unstable surface) helps improve spinal alignment. It reduces the tendency of slouching. It also makes upright sitting much easier and more comfortable.

By gently recruiting the stabilizing multifidus, proprioceptive sitting helps prevent the stiffening and the persistent contraction of these muscles. Over time it also helps to exercise and strengthen these muscles and to stabilize and strengthen the lower back as well as improve core stability.

By activating gentle imbibition processes to spinal discs (hydration of the spinal discs, either naturally or through treatment), proprioceptive sitting helps improve hydration to spinal discs.

While sitting on an unstable surface, you must start with a low level of instability and short durations of stimulation that is about 30-minutes per episode for most people. You can repeat such stimulation multiple times throughout the day, and gradually prolong the time in which you sit on the unstable surface. It generally takes about three months of gradual extension of the time of sitting on a gently unstable surface, until you would sit on it throughout the day.

This is the key to
1. Help maintain focus on your work, especially in an office
2. Help prevent overwork of your back muscles.

It is not correct for people to start with sitting on a stability ball the whole day at work, because it will lead to back fatigue while leading to poor posture and unexpected damage to the back.

3. The Loosening Nature of the Soft Tissues

The ligaments and muscles around your spine are similar to the clothes around your body. They need to snugly fit with your spine's skeletal structure to allow it to function properly.

However, they are not completely like a rubber band and can't immediately return to their original size and shape after being stretched for a prolonged period.

As a result, they become loose temporarily, and affect the function of the spine, while you are getting on with your daily activities. Imagine how it might feel to you if the waist of your pants suddenly became a few sizes bigger while you were jogging. This loosening nature is scientifically known as the "viscoelastic nature."

Viscoelastic nature is a material process of both viscosity and elasticity-type behaviours when the spine is under stress.

Viscosity behaviour allows the material to deform with lasting effect, if the stress is applied long enough. While elasticity allows the material to regain its original form.

With viscosity at play, the material will not be able to regain its original form completely, once, after a period of time, outside stress is relieved.

Studies have shown all soft connective tissues including muscles, tendons, and ligaments are viscoelastic. It means that your muscles, tendons, and ligaments will not be able to regain their original shape, form, length, strength or balance, once the outside stress disappears. The outside stress needs a minimum period to be able to activate the viscosity response in the soft tissues.

This is why you must stretch for a long period of time if you want to increase your range of motion. To achieve the best results, you need to stretch for more than 20-minutes. At the same time, this is also why your muscles, tendons, and ligaments will not be negatively affected by the short stretches in your daily activities and exercises, which typically last about 30-seconds - not long enough for the viscosity property of your soft tissues to work.

However, this nature of the body may also work against you. If your postural muscles, tendons, and ligaments are incorrectly stretched, they may become undesirably loose, which makes it difficult to keep up a healthy posture.

Slouching while sitting is one of the most pervasive activities in which undesirable stretches of your back muscles, tendons, and ligaments take place, because sitting typically lasts a prolonged period which allows the viscosity nature of the soft tissues to work.

As a result, slouched sitting invariably leads to or reinforces further poor posture, because your muscles, tendons, and ligaments around your spine are loosened, like the waist length of your pants is suddenly increased by two sizes.

This nature affects the entire biomechanics of your back and body. The health of the viscoelastic nature of your back muscles, tendons, and ligaments is critical to the health of your back.

A study shows that muscles lose their resistance capacity after being stretched five times for only 90-seconds each time.

The study created a viscoelastic response of a person's hamstring muscle and found after each 90-second stretch, it became less resistant to each stretch. The stretches were repeated five times.

Static stretching decreases the viscosity of tendon structures while increasing the elasticity. This provides a physiological background for reducing passive resistance and improving joint range of motion after stretching. In the case of our posture, this translates into a slouched back.

4. The Inside-out Nature of the Body

Our body is an integrated whole. Issues in one part of the body often lead to symptoms and issues in other parts of the body. Issues with inner organs may show symptoms on the outside of the body. This inside-out nature is medically known as a "viscerosomatic reflex."

Viscerosomatic reflex is a connective nature of our body, in which internal organs are connected to other corresponding parts neurologically. It is an inside-out nature of our body. Viscerosomatic reflex occurs when a diseased internal organ transmits signals to the brain.

Once reaching the spinal cord, this signal gets relayed and expressed in other body parts. From the spinal cord onwards, the pain signals from inner organs and related outer body parts use the same ascending nerve channel (interneuron).

As a result any irritation signal sent by the inner organ could be interpreted by the brain as an irritation signal from the related outer body part, leading the brain to perceive the corresponding outer body part as suffering from irritation or pain.

This could create the perception that all body parts on the same sensory channel of the spinal cord are experiencing pain as a result of pain felt in the soft tissues of any of such body parts. For example, a heart attack can cause chest and/or left arm pain in the sufferer.

In particular, there is a strong connection between your back and the inner organs in your thoracic, abdominal, and pelvic cavities, including these cavities themselves. Problems in inner organs often manifest themselves as pain in the back. Typical examples are: lower back pain caused by menstruation, ovary issues, uterus problems, kidney infection/kidney stones, bleeding/infection in the pelvis, or lower back or sciatic pain from severe constipation.

Cancer also often creates pain in the back, such as pancreatic cancer causing pain in the lower back, and lung cancer causing pain in the mid to upper back. For example, lung cancer may irritate nerves traveling through the chest or the lining of the lungs, which can be interpreted by the brain as back pain.

Similar to viscerosomatic reflex – where what happens on the inside of our body can affect the outside -- the reverse is also true. There is also a "somatoviscero reflex" nature in our body – where what happens on the outside of our body can affect the inside. It is an outside-in nature of body.

This nature is often used by manual medicine to reach and treat the inner organs with external body parts. The most typical examples are acupuncture, massage, chiropractic, osteopath, and reflexology. This nature makes it possible to treat your back pain, even when the pain is from an inner organ instead of your back directly. Of course, this somatoviscero reflex nature is used to help our body in ways far more than merely treating back pain.

Points of learning of viscerosomato nature of the body are twofold.

First, back pain may not necessarily mean that there is something wrong with your back. Your back pain may be an indication of something wrong elsewhere in your body.

Second, back pain is not to be taken lightly because it may be an indicator for a far more serious problem in your body. It is critical to diagnose it properly to find out its true cause or at least rule out the risk of serious illness.

Don't fool yourself by using drugs, ice packs or pain creams to cover it up. You may lose valuable time and a window of opportunity in attacking the more severe illness early on. An ounce of prevention is worth a pound of cure. In the same principle, one week of early treatment may be worth more than one year of delayed care.

5. The Emotional Nature of Back Pain
It has been widely studied and proven that emotional and mental stress can cause pain in the back. As a result, the origin of your back pain may not only be outside of your back, but also beyond your

inner organs.

According to a Quebec study, relationship stress can be closely related to back pain. And in 1984, Dr. John Sarno introduced the concept of Tension Myositis Syndrome (TMS) to back pain caused by physiological alternation in certain muscles, nerves, tendons, and ligaments due to emotional stress. Dr. Sarno found the muscles most susceptible to TMS are the postural muscles in the lower back and neck. That is why emotional stress can cause back pain.

The bad news is that we are living in a high pressure and high stress society. Our average perceived levels of stress are between 7- to 8 on a scale from 1 to 10, with 10 as the highest level of stress. Most people suffer some emotional and mental stress.

The good news is that emotional and mental stress is to a large degree, if not completely, controllable with most people. There are many techniques and exercises to help you keep your emotional and mental stress in check. You may wish to participate in stress reducing activities, such as Yoga, Tai Chi, meditation, getting out and enjoying nature, playing with pets, playing music, swimming, painting and so on.

Staying positive while avoiding negative situations that cause stress may cause the distraction you need to forget about your back pain. Look on the upside. See the glass as half full. Lighten your heart. Be more humorous. Be with your friends more. Get social support. Watch a comedy. Do more things you enjoy. Stay away from people, activities, and environments that upset you.

You may also want to smile and laugh more. Express your feelings instead of bottling them up. Even talking to strangers will make you feel better and happier. Look at the big picture. Compromise more. Adapt yourself more to people and the environment around you. View things from other people's perspective more. Stay away from arguing the unarguable. Trying to win in a conflict will create a lot of stress on yourself. Your winning may also mean another person's "loss" that will come back and bite you. Take breaks from stressful situations. Take timeouts. Forgive others, events, and environment more. Avoid controlling the uncontrollable.

Here's what you need to know about the emotional nature of back pain – it is twofold.

First, keep a calm mind. Take care of yourself. Don't distress yourself with anything unnecessarily. Don't sweat the small stuff.

Second, develop skills to control and manage your emotions.

6. The Vulnerable Nature of the Spine

Our spine carries our body weight, supports our body balance, and facilitates our body's motion. It takes every twist and turn of our body. It suffers wear and tear over time. It puts up with the shocks and dehydration with every step we take. It deals with the degeneration of the discs and vertebrae. As a result, out spine is one of the more vulnerable parts of our body.

The most mobile sections of the spine, such as the lower back and the neck, are where most back injuries and pains occur.

The lower the disc or vertebrae in the spine, the higher the body weight it bears. For example, the vertebra on the very top of the spine only needs to support the weight of the head. The vertebrae at the base of the neck will have to support both the head and the neck. In the same principle, the lowest lumbar vertebrae or disc will have to take on the weight of the head, the neck, the arms and hands, and the most of the trunk.

Luckily, the vertebrae and discs are thicker and bigger as they go down the spine, to take on this greater load. Unfortunately, this is still not sufficient because of other factors at play.

Also, our spine has to support the balance of our body. In this case, the vertebrae or disc in the spine works like a pivot. The spine could only be in a balanced and stable condition, if the loads on the pivot are balanced out. This leads to naturally increased load on the vertebrae or discs because the spine not only has to take the weight but also the extra load to balance the asymmetry of that weight.

Take the middle disc in the lumbar spine for an example. This disc functions as a pivot point to two counter acting loads.

The first load is the body weight, whose gravity center is slightly forward of the center of the disc when the person is standing still.

The second load is a force created by the muscles behind the spine to counter balance the first load. The center of this force is roughly in an equal distance to the center of the spinal disc, compared with the gravity center of the upper body weight above this disc. Because this force adds to the upper body weight to form the total load on the disc, we could call it a phantom weight – it functions like a weight, but is not a weight.

Based on the Law of Moments according to which the sum of the clockwise moments is equal to the sum of the anticlockwise moments when an object is balanced (in equilibrium), the force (PWb) generated by the back muscles in this case shall equal to the upper body weight (Wb) – the weight of the body part above the horizontal level of the spinal disc that needs to bear said upper body weight, because the distance between the centre of the spinal disc in the lower back and the gravity center line of the upper body (DWb) roughly equals the distance between the centre of the spinal disc in the lower back and the stabilizing muscles (DPW) when human body is in a upright position, and clockwise moment PWb x DPW shall

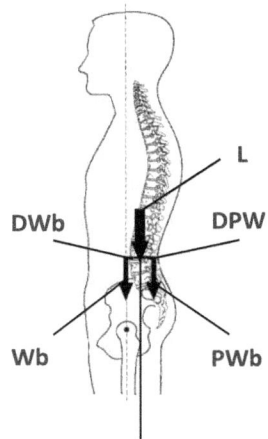

Source: Patrick Lee

Fig. 1.4

equal the counter clockwise moment Wb x DWb. As a result, the total load (L) on the spinal disc shall be twice the upper body wright - L = Wb + PWb.

If the weight of the upper body including the head, neck, arms, and hands is 80 LB, the counter balancing force in the muscles is also 80 LB. Because both the weight and the muscle force points downward, the actual load on the disc is 160 LB, double that of the body weight above the level of the disc.

Similarly, if you have a heavy weight in your hands, the total load on your spinal disc will far exceed the sum of your upper body weight and the weight you carry, because of are two instead of one phantom weights your spine has to take – the Handling Weight which is an force in the back muscle to balance the weight you lift, and the Postural Weight which is a force in the back muscles to balance your body weight.

A Postural Weight is determined by your body weight and your posture. Handling Weight is determined by the way you lift or carry the external weight, such as you list a heavy suitcase, a large pot of flowers, a garbage bin, a crate of beer, a bag of deicing salt, or a child close to and far away from your body.

The four weights your lower spine takes are:

- Wb – the weight of your body above the level of the vertebra or disc measured

- We – the external weigh you lift or carry

- PWb – phantom weight your spine takes due to your own body biomechanics and posture

- PWe – phantom weight your spine takes due to the way you lift or carry external weight.

- DWb – the distance between the centre of the spinal disc in the lower back and the gravity center line of the upper body.

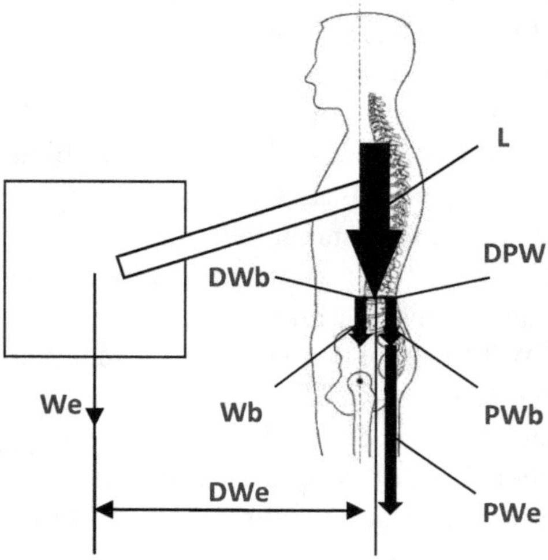

Source: Patrick Lee
Fig. 1.5

- DWe – the horizontal distance between the centre of the spinal disc in the lower back and the centre of your load-bearing hand which shall roughly be aligned with the gravity center line of the weight you lift.

- DPW – the distance between the centre of the spinal disc in the lower back and the stabilizing muscles.

PWb = Wb*DWb/DPW

PWe = We*DWe/DPW

L = (Wb + PWb) + (We + PWe)

DWb varies with your posture. While standing, DWb roughly equals DPW. As a result PWb roughly equals Wb. However, when you sit, DWb often increases to 1.5 to 2 DPW, which cause the PWb to increase to 1.5 to 2 times of Wb. When you slouch while sitting,

DWb further increases to 3-5 times of DPW, which means that PWb will be 3-5 times of Wb.

DWb also varies with your body structure and condition. In the case of women with prominent breasts or men with a prominent belly, DWb, hence PWb, will significantly increase.

DWe varies with your way of handling the external weight. When external weight is kept close to your body, such as when you carry a briefcase at your side or carry a child on your shoulders, DWe would be as low as 1 time of DPW. As a result PWe would equal 1 time of We. However, if you lift the same child with your arms stretched out, DWe could increase up to 28-30 times of DPW, which causes the PWe to jump up to 28-30 times of We.

This means, if you let the 30 LB child sit on your shoulders, the stress in your back muscles could be just 30 LB, and the total additional load on your spinal disc shall be only 60 LB. However, if you hold a 30 LB child with your arms fully stretched out, the stress in your back muscles could be as high as 900 LB, and the total additional load on your spinal disc shall be 930 LB – a 15 fold increase in the total additional load on your spinal discs. The total additional load your spine has to take is far more than the external weight alone. How are you going to carry your child or lift a heavy weight the next time? What are you going to do the next time when there is a risk that your body weight may exceed a healthy level?

If you stand up right and carry no external weight, the total spinal load = (Wb + PWb) + (We + PWe)
= 2x Wb (because DWb = DPW)
= 2 times the total upper body weight

If you you stand up right and carry an external weight (that weighs one half of your upper body weight) on your shoulders, the total spinal load = (Wb + PWb) + (We + PWe)
= 2x Wb + 2x We (because DWe = DPW and DWb = DPW)
= 3x Wb
= 3 times the total upper body weight

If you you stand up right and carry an external weight (that weighs one half of your upper body weight) in your hands with your arms fully stretched out, the total spinal load = (Wb + PWb) + (We + PWe)

= 2x Wb + 31We (because DWe = 30 DPW, and DWb = DPW)

= 17.5x Wb

= 17.5 times of the total upper body weight

The difference between the minimum and maximum load is merely in how close the external weight is kept to your body and whether you bend your body forward or not. (Note: if you take and hold a big breath while doing the lifting, the load your spine has to take dramatically declines. More on this in Part Three, Chapter 1, Section 4 "Use Your Legs and Breath, not Your Back" of this book.

As a result, the phantom weight your spine has to take on significantly exceeds the sum of your body weight and external weight.

Since phantom weight is significantly and easily affected by your posture and your way of handling the external weight, you have every reason to maintain a good posture and use the right way to handle your external weight.

The lower back is one of the most sensitive parts of the spine or back because it takes on most of the load of the body and most of the load that we carry externally in our daily activities. Almost every mobile activity we engage in requires the facilitation of the lower back. To lift a child, we have to bend our back forward (in the sagittal plane in which we move our body front and back). To look up overhead and reach up high, we often bend it backward. To turn our body around, we need to rotate our lumbar area clockwise or counter clockwise (in the axial plane). And we often need to bend our spine to the left or right side ways (in the coronal plane).

Our spinal discs give us the ability to rotate and bend when needed. Spinal discs are the soft links between our vertebrae and allow the flexibility of our spine. Because of the countless motions put on them, they are subjected to wear and tear.

The sensitivity of the neck is also determined by further characteristics of the neck, other than forward head posture. The neck is the thinnest and weakest part of the spine. The cross section of a vertebra in the neck is generally only one quarter of those in the lower back. Yet, the neck is responsible for even more bending, twisting and turning. For each bending, twisting or turning of the back, there is a 10-fold bending, twisting or turning in the neck. In other words, the neck is used 10-times more than the lower back.

The neck is also the least supported portion of the spine. Besides the rather thin muscles around the cervical spine, there is nothing else to support or protect it, far less than the back which has chest, abdomen and pelvis as reinforcements. For example, in auto accidents, the first and most frequent injury suffered is whiplash in the neck.

Whiplash occurs when a passenger's head is hurled backwards and then forward violently. This often happens when one car is hit in the rear by another. Whiplash can occur at a relative low speed of 24 kilometers per hour (that's fifteen miles per hour) or less. Whiplash can harm the nerves, muscles, discs and vertebrae in the neck. The higher the relative speed, and the more sudden the thrust motion, the more bones, discs, muscles and tendons in the neck and upper back will be damaged. The resulting pain can last a few weeks to several months. About a quarter of all cases may develop into chronic pain and lasting disability that may have long term effects throughout the person's life and work. In the U.S. 5,000 whiplash injuries result in quadriplegia each year.

Whiplash is one of the main injuries covered by automobile insurance. According to National Highway Traffic Safety Administration (NHTSA), there are approximately 806,000 occupants that sustain whiplash injuries in motor vehicle crashes in the United States each year. The majority of cases occur in people in their late 40s. Such injuries are responsible for a significant portion of every driver's insurance premium.

In the split second of a car accident, many things happen and may determine your fate for the rest of your life.

Within one second, the fine vertebrae, disc, muscles and tendons in the neck suffer more violent abuse than most of their peers in the middle or lower spine would experience in a life time, all without any support.

Our spine, especially the neck and lumbar area, is vulnerable, which is proven by the fact that 80 percent of all North Americans will experience an acute episode of back pain in their lives and by the fact that $200 Billion is spent directly on treating back pain each year in the US alone.

Some people may try to convince you that your spine is the

strongest structure in your body. This may be true from a point of view that a spine rarely falls apart or is fully broken. However, not falling apart or not being fully broken is not an adequate benchmark for today's expected quality of life. While rarely falling apart, the spine does often malfunction and lead to back pain compromising bodily functions and limiting bodily range of motion and freedom.

However, vulnerability doesn't justify fear. What it does justify, even calls for, is our attention to taking preventative measures for our spine. We must see this vulnerability the way it is. To ignore this vulnerability, for the sake of avoiding fear, is not the right way to go. No one should take the back for granted, even irresponsibly abuse it, and subject it to severe trauma, repetitive strains, poor posture or subject it to still sitting at work for many hours in a row, or stuff it in a car seat for hundreds of miles without proper support, or subject it to sudden motion without giving it a chance to warm up. After all, had our spine not been taken for granted, back pain wouldn't have been so pervasive in this world. Any advice telling you your back or spine is strong and not vulnerable is questionable.

7. The Self-Enforcing Nature of Poor Posture
The leaning tower of Pisa, Italy is world famous. While the included posture of the tower is pleasing to the eyes, it is extremely hard for the foundation that holds it up. As a result, the incline of the tower continue to increase over time. Without urgent measures, the tower will collapse in the not too distant future, because the further the tower inclines, the harder it becomes for the foundation to hold the tower up, which leads to increased incline and increased difficulty for the foundation to hold the tower up.

While this self-reinforcing vicious circle happens to the posture of a building, it also happens to the posture of the human body, especially if you have forward head posture (FHP), a hunched back, and or slouch a lot.

Of course, more factors are at play in the case of human posture. Among other factors, the self-reinforcing neuro-patterning of the body and the viscoelastic nature of the soft tissues makes the self-reinforcing nature of the poor posture more viscous and difficult to correct than in the case of a building.

Our neck is in an especially difficult situation in modern life. Fact is that with every inch of forward protrusion of the head, the stress in the neck muscles that hold the head up increases by 100 percent. Figuratively speaking, you would be adding an extra head on your shoulders (which weighs approximately 10 LB, like an average watermelon) with each inch of forward protrusion of your head. Knowingly and unknowingly, people often lean their head 1 to 3 inches forward, which means that they are carrying 1 to 3 extra heads, each one of which equals a 10 LB watermelon, on their shoulders. Imagine what a horrible punishment it is to be forced to carry three 10 LB watermelons on your shoulders, 24 hours a day, 365 days a year!

Unfortunately, these extra heads do not give you any additional brain power. In all likelihood, they tend to reduce your existing brain power by consuming more of your physical and mental energy when you carry these dead weights around. Furthermore, the nagging neck pains and headaches that these extra weights and associated poor posture often cause actually cuts your mental focus and brain power by a magnitude you don't want to imagine. Just think about the level of your mental power or focus you had when you suffered headaches the last time.

In our past, our head position was mostly up and facing forward. Unfortunately, in today's life, our head is mostly tilted forward and face down. Simply take some time to observe the people around you and you will quickly find that their heads are down most of the time, from office workers working at their computers, to children doing homework, to moms preparing food in the kitchen, to seniors doing their craft work, to people reading a book, writing a text on a smart phone, playing a game on an iPad, even commuters driving a car to work. If you track the time from the first thing in the morning, such as brushing your teeth, to the last thing you do before sleep, such as watching TV in bed, you may realize that about 80 percent of the time your head is leaned forward.

8. The Pervasive Nature of Spinal Degeneration

Spinal degeneration is an inescapable natural process. In fact, it is a part of our aging process. Talking about aging, most people think about the lines on their face, the bags under their eyes, or the sagging of their chin. Most people spend hundreds, if not thousands, of dollars on cosmetics a year to take care of the face, their outer beauty. However, few people pay enough attention to their spine – the source of their inner beauty. Most people start to think of it often when the damage is already done and requires huge financial resources to slow it down, if at all possible.

Of course, understandably, the inner beauty is way more important than the outer beauty, because it has a far greater impact on your health, wellbeing, and happiness.

Think of your spine as the frame of a house. Would you prefer your house to have a burned and rotten frame with a front door covered by a layer of fresh paint? Do you think such a house be able to withstand any storms or minor earthquake? Would you dare to live inside it? Or, would you prefer your house to have a strong and solid frame but a few little spots of rust on the front door? I am sure that you will choose the latter 10 out of 10 times.

Think of your spine as the frame of your house, and treat it accordingly. Take care of its substance before worrying about the cosmetic appearance. Remember, the smile of your back is hundred times more important than the clothes on your back or the glow on your face. In fact, if your back is mad, your face can't possibly have a glow on it.

For each dollar you spend on your cosmetics, you need to spend at least one dollar on your spine and back. Otherwise you are literally spending time on painting your front door instead of taking care of the frame of your house, while it may be rotting away.

Believe or not, the degeneration of your spine starts as early as 19 years of age. At the age of 19, the self lubrication function of your spinal discs stops.

The second major cause of spinal degeneration is bone absorption process. In your early years, your body creates more bone material than it absorbs. However, this changes around the age of 30 when your body begins to absorb more bone material than it creates. This process accelerates for women when their estrogen production slows down around 45 – 55, and for men when their testosterone begins to decline around age of 45-50.

Besides the natural degeneration, that takes place solely due to aging, there is also a behavioral degeneration that is caused by:

- A sedentary lifestyle
- Poor use of the back
- Being overweight
- Smoking

- Poor diet
- Illness, or
- Medication.

Spinal degeneration can lead to the following issues:
• Stiffness of the back.
• Discomfort or pain after long periods of still sitting or standing.
• Difficulty getting up from a sitting position.
• Decreased range of bending and twisting motion in the spine.
• Risk of back problems increases as weather gets cold
• Increased sensitivity to stress in the spine.
• Increased risk of spinal fracture in minor trauma.
• Prolonged period to recover from any back or spinal injury.
• Increased risk of disc dehydration.
• Increased risk of spinal nerves being pinched.
• Increased risk of osteoarthritis.
• Increased risk of spinal stenosis.

Unfortunately, like a mechanical part that does not lubricate itself, for most of a person's life, the discs need to be properly lubricated and taken care of.

Fortunately, most of the lubrication is done subconsciously through the various physical activities we conduct in our daily lives.

The lubrication of our discs works like a clam under the sea. It opens its shells and fresh water goes in. As they close, the stale water gets pushed out. Our discs get lubricated with each bending motion of the spine. When the spine bends in whichever direction, the space between two vertebrae gets opened like a clam opens its shells, and fresh nutritious body fluid gets drawn into the space that is occupied by the discs that sucks the fresh fluid like a sponge. When the spine returns to its straight condition, the intervertebral spaces get closed and the old fluid gets squeezed out. This process is often referred to as the imbibition process.

What if we stand or sit still for a prolonged period? Our spinal discs will dehydrate and compress. Since our spinal bending action is not in existence, the clam-like opening and closing of our intervertebral spaces cease to exist. Our spinal discs cease to receive new fresh nutritious and lubricating fluid. And at the same time, the constant body weight that is placed on the discs slowly squeezes out the fluid that was in the disc before. Due to the increasing weight load on the discs as they move down the spine, the discs in the lower spine are mostly affected by this process, and most likely to be dehydrated due to their sponge like nature.

What if we sit in front of a computer or TV for prolonged period? Our discs dehydrate, compress, ligaments in the back stretch and fatigue, and back muscles are deprived of blood supply.

What happens if you suddenly need to move to pick up something from the ground? Your dehydrated spine discs will be forced to jump into action. Forcing discs to work without lubricating fluid is like starting an engine without engine oil. They will suffer extra wear and tear and they may "burn" in your spine leading to back pain or injury.

Speed of this dehydration process increases as spinal degeneration progresses, which often happen as we age. As a result, a child or a young person may be able to sit or stand still for prolonged periods, such as the famed Scottish Guards in front of Buckingham Palace, because it takes longer for their spinal discs to dehydrate.

But older people will experience unexpected consequences when doing so, because their spinal discs are faster to lose fluid without imbibition. As a result, from a spinal biomechanics point of view, older people need to move more than younger people. Unfortunately, the reality is exactly the opposite. However, this should at least serve as a reminder or warning to our senior fellow citizens, you need to move, not just your fingers, but your back. Sitting and swinging your legs is not sufficient to prevent dehydration.

9. The Increase of Pain Sensors with Age

Our spinal disc has a shape of an ice hockey puck that has three major parts – a round cookie like jelly core (nucleus), cylindrical side wall (annulus) and flat endplates on top and bottoms of the disc.
The cylindrical wall is made of 10-20 layers of belt like thin walls (lamellae). The thin walls pile up together to make a thick and strong disc wall of about 10 mm in thickness. The outer one third of a healthy disc wall is wired with nerves (nociceptors) that can transmit pain signals.

These nerves are sensitive to excessive pressure and deformation. Under abnormal pressure, stress, or injury in the discs, these pain receptors will be activated and send out pain signals to the brain and cause the body to feel pain in the back. Such pains are often centralized in the disc, and referred to as discogenic pain which is often overlooked in back pain treatments.

Dehydrated and degenerated spinal discs become denser and thinner, which often leads to increased squeezing and pressure on the pain receptors, which then may fire and lead to pain in the back.

On the other hand, according to Spanish researcher José García-Cosamalón and his co-authors, as a person ages or experiences spinal degeneration, her or his spinal discs shrink and the nociceptors experience a renewed growth spurt. As a result, the degenerated spinal discs become more densely populated with nociceptors (more densely innervated) even in regions that in normal conditions lack population of nociceptors (innervation). Such increased population of nerves is linked with increased senilities towards stress and tension in the back and increased instances of back pain amongst seniors, as one of the leading causes.

As a result of the combined effects of the above two phenomenon, senior citizens are more likely to feel back pain by nature, when all other factors are equal. This is a good self-protective nature of the body. It helps seniors to slow down a bit, and to be a little more careful with their body, to protect their body and back.

The downside of this good nature is that it also tends to lead to reduced involvement in physical activities, which is detrimental to the health of their back. Seniors need to consciously be aware of this nature and push themselves to be engaged in moderate physical activities frequently.

10. Sitting is the New Smoking

Your body is built to move, not to remain still, for the very need of basic self-survival. However, sedentary lifestyles increasingly tie people to their chairs and reduce their physical activities. Physical inactivity is more prevalent than obesity. In America, one in three may have obesity, but more than one in two is insufficiently engaged in physical activities. Physical inactivity leads to increased inflammation, change in metabolism, change in blood circulation, change in blood pressure, contributes to anxiety and depression, coronary heart disease, high cholesterol, diabetes, cancer (especially breast cancer and colon cancer), obesity, and premature death.

Sitting is the new smoking, both from the perspective of its health damage and its pervasiveness. The physical inactivity of sitting has long been linked with a large number of health problems far beyond back pain alone. Such health issues range from obesity to cardiovascular diseases. A recent study by the American Institute for Cancer Research has found the physical inactivity of sitting is also linked with several common cancers - 25 percent of colon cancer and 28 percent of breast cancers are due to sitting.

While you need to increase your engagement in general physical activities, you also need to maintain movement in your body, especially in your back, during stationary activities, such as sitting in an office, working on a computer, watching TV or movies, reading a book, traveling in cars, buses, trains, boats or on airplanes.

"You must be kidding! Should I keep moving around while sleeping too?" you may say. No, you don't. The reason is that keeping movement in your back is only important when your back is working against gravity. Your back works against gravity when you sit, stand, walk, run, and do sports. However, your back doesn't work against gravity when you sleep.

Why does gravity make such a big difference? It is an evolutional nature, that when your back works against gravity, tension builds up in your back muscles, especially the deep stabilizing muscles. In our discussion about the tensegrity nature of the back, we discussed that what holds your back upright is not your spine, but your back muscles. Your spine only plays a passive role in this process. It is your deep stabilizing muscles that are playing an active role in pulling and keeping your back upright.

Under static tension when there is no movement in your back, your deep stabilizing muscles tend to stiffen and contract 20-minutes after the static tension begins. Such stiffening and contracting processes of the muscles compromise blood flow to the muscles, increases waste remaining in the muscles that often result in muscle pain and fatigue. The stiffening and contracting process of deep stabilizing muscles also increases the pressure on spinal discs. Since spinal discs have pain receptors that respond to excess pressure and deformation, the increased pressure on spinal discs may also fire pain signals causing back pain.

Keep as much movement in your back as you comfortably can, whenever your back is working against gravity, i.e. in an upright position, whether you are sitting or standing.

How do you keep movements in your back while sitting or standing?

For sitting, use an unstable sitting foundation. There are many chairs, seat cushions, discs, and balls developed for this purpose. You need to pay attention to the level of instability a particular chair, seat cushion, disc or ball provides. The higher level of instability such devices offer, the more physical activities will be invoked in your back. Too high a level of physical activity stimulated in your back should be used for short durations only, because it may be distractive to you from your work, and may also be overtly challenging to your body.

For prolonged sitting, especially for use in the office or in any situation where you need to focus your attention on certain tasks, such as working on a computer, a low level of stimulation is desirable. The right level of stimulation tends to be a level at which your mind does not have to think about balancing your body, and can comfortably focus on your task on hand.

Since every individual is different, and every sitting situation is different, it may be desirable and practical to use a device whose level of seating instability can be easily adjusted and customized. In fact, easy customizability of the neuromuscular stimulation needs to be a key criteria when purchasing your next chair or seating device.

2

Why It Is The Cause That You Must Treat?

Back pain is a bodily sensation that refers to a wide range of unpleasant sensory and emotional experiences associated with actual or potential tissue, skeletal or inner organ damage. Pain is a warning signal transmitted from pain receptors to our brain, through the spinal cord, with its intensity proportional to the level of actual or potential damage to our body.

Back pain is an alarm signal perceived in the back but it's origin may be far beyond the confines of your back. Back pain is not an illness. It is merely an alarm signal telling you that something may be wrong with your back, with your inner organs or with your emotional or mental state. Your treatments need to focus on the cause instead of the signals themselves, unless your alarm system malfunctions, which, fortunately, happens exceedingly rarely with your back.

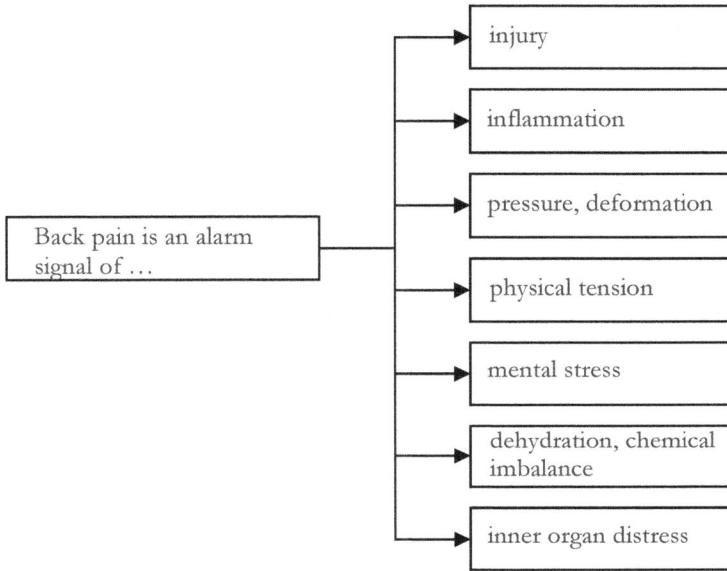

Source: compiled by Patrick Lee

Fig. 1.6

Most ailments of the body cause pain. Pain travels through three redundant pathways to the brain, to protect our body, to minimize tissue or skeletal injury. Individuals insensitive to pain tend to be injured badly. Being able to experience pain is critical to our health, wellbeing, even survival.

Spinothalamic tract: The information transmitted via this tract is regarded as affective sensation, such a sensation is accompanied by a compulsion to act. For instance, an itch is accompanied by an urge to scratch, and a burning stimulus makes us automatically withdraw from the heat source. In the spinal cord, the Spinothalamic tract originates two additional sensory tracts – the Paleospinothalamic tract and the Neospinothalamic tract – to reach different parts of the brain and to make sure that pain signals will be received by the brain. This is nature's redundancy design which came millions of years ahead of the modern day redundancy designed in our internet and digital world

Paleospinothalamic tract: This tract transmits the signal of a diffuse ache that is motivational-affective, meaning it does not allow exact localization, but alerts the body it is hurt and needs to react immediately to avoid further damage.

Neospinothalamic tract: This tract transmits signals of fast pain allowing for perception of different shades of pain and permitting localization of the pain. Fast pain is felt within a tenth of a second of application of the pain stimulus and is a sharp, acute, prickling pain felt in response to mechanical and thermal stimulation. This is the signal that allows one to withdraw her hand when in contact with a hot plate.

Most back pain is the result of trivial matters, such as bending down to pick up a pencil from the floor or waking up with back pain after a night of sleep. And most of these can be prevented.

According to Dr. Randy A. Shelerund, MD, Director of Spine Center, Mayo Clinic, very few visits to the Mayo Clinic for back pain have been because of traumatic injury or heavy weight lifting. The pinching on the nerves exiting the spine or on the spinal cord is often a critical cause for back pain. Inadequate appreciation of this fact is often the cause for failure of medical intervention.

Back muscles, ligaments, tendons, fascia have within them nerve endings (nociceptors, or painreceptors) capable of transmitting pain impulses. These nerve endings are sensitive to stretching, tearing, pressure, etc. Nociceptors were discovered by Charles Scott Sherrington in 1906 who also discovered proprioceptors and the proprioceptive nature of our body.

There are five types of nociceptors by their sensitivities towards:

1. Mechanical pressure or deformation, e.g. cuts, tears, impacts, fractures, etc.
2. Chemical stimulation, e.g. metabolites from traumatized tissues, such as arachidonic acid and prostaglandins, or inflammatory chemicals.
3. Thermal extremes, e.g. burning sensation.
4. Actual injury, although each nociceptor has different sensitivity threshold levels, some do not respond at all to chemical, thermal or mechanical stimuli unless injury or inflammation actually has occurred. These are referred to as silent nociceptors.
5. Multiple stimuli, many receptors respond to more than one stimuli, instead of one single stimuli, such as thermal, mechanical, and chemical stimuli. Often referred to as

polymodal receptors.

Strong stimuli may trigger reflex withdrawal, autonomic responses, such as increased heart rate, heightened blood pressure, and intensified respiration, along with pain, for self-protective purposes. Interestingly, in the presence of pain and the support of various neuropeptides, the sensitivities of such nociceptors change to such an extent where normal physiological pressure changes often lead to strong and chronic firing of these receptors, hence triggering pain . This explains why some people experience strong or chronic pain with no mechanical irritation to the nervous system, nor with any temperature or chemical irritation, commonly known as phantom pain.

Back pain due to nerve interference may happen when the spine is not properly aligned or when one or more spinal discs significantly deforms, such as in the case of disc hernia. In a misaligned spine, vertebrae are dislocated in relation to each other, which often leads to change of the narrow nerve pathway between the vertebrae. Such change often means narrowing of the nerve pathway, which may result in corresponding nerves being compressed or jammed by the dislocated vertebrae. Misalignment of the spine often happens when a person stands, sits, works or sleeps in a poor posture.

While most back pains are mechanical in nature, a minority of back pains are associated with inflammatory conditions, such as arthritis. Such inflammatory back pains often have symptoms, such as:

- A slow onset over a period of three months or more.
- Worsening with rest
- In the morning often accompanied with stiffness lasting 30-minutes or more.
- Improving with exercise
- Improving with anti-inflammatory drugs (e.g. ibuprofen).

Back pain often begins as tingling sensation in the deep and fine stabilizing muscles, i.e. muscles closest to the spine, and gradually intensifies and spreads out.

Back pain is your body's way of telling you something is wrong with your back or spine, or some part of the back or spine is not functioning properly, and attention is required.

In most cases, a pain itself is not the problem, but only the signal of one or more problems. Hence, when back pain happens, one needs to pay attention to the underlying cause instead of the pain itself. Pain killers can only cut off the pain signal to your brain, but they do not heal or take away the cause. If the underlying issue is not resolved, back pain will continue regardless if you feel it or not. The fact that your brain does not sense a pain, does not mean that the pain or problem is not there or that the problem has been resolved. One should only take pain killers with a clear understanding of this fact and continue to identify the cause to reduce and prevent your back pain.

There are many types of back pain; however, over 90 percent of them are mechanical in nature -- caused by a mechanical disorder of back muscles, ligaments, nerves, spinal discs and vertebrae. Such mechanical back pains are caused mostly by lifting things or performing repetitive activities that are challenging to the back, and are often associated with certain occupations, such as:

- Nursing;
- Construction workers;
- Dentists;
- Mining workers;
- Mechanics repairing vehicles, engines, heavy machineries;
- Sedentary workers, such as office workers, call center workers, as sitting has become the leading cause for back pain and injury second only to heavy weight lifting.

According to the American Academy of Orthopaedic Surgeons (AAOS), 30 percent of American adults are afflicted by back pain each year. And an astounding 50 percent of American working adults are afflicted by back pain in any given year, according to Alf Nachemson, MD, PhD. A study published in *Spine* in 2003 even indicates that 25 percent of all adults are affected by lower back pain in any given month.

Fortunately, 60 to -70 percent of people with back pain recover in six weeks and 80 to 90 percent of them recover in 12-weeks. After 12-weeks, further natural recovery is slow.

Furthermore, 5 to 10 percent of all lower back pain becomes chronic after initial onset. Twenty to forty percent of back pain episodes are likely to reoccur within one year. As high as 85 percent of back pain sufferers will endure recurring back pain after the initial episode in their lifetime.

Back pain may be constant or intermittent, acute or chronic, concentrated in one area or radiating to other parts of the body, mechanical or inflammatory, with a dull or sharp sensation, with a tingling or a numb feeling.

Based on the location, back pain can be divided into:

- Neck pain,
- Upper back pain,
- Mid back pain,
- Lower back pain,
- Sacrum pain (Sacrum is the triangular bone at the back of the spine), and
- Tailbone pain.

Based on duration, back pain can be categorized into acute pain that lasts up to 6-weeks, chronic pain that lasts more than 12-weeks, and subacute pain that lasts 6 to 12-weeks.

Based on cause, back pain can be categorized into specific and nonspecific back pain.

Specific back pains are the pains whose causes can be clearly identified. Specific back pains include:

- Degenerative back pain,
- Inflammatory back pain,
- Infectious back pain,
- Neuroplastic back pain,
- Traumatic back pain,
- Deformative back pain,
- Neurogenic back pain, and
- Congenital back pain.

Nonspecific back pains are pains whose cause can't be clearly identified. According to Dr. Shane Burch of University of California, nonspecific back pains represent 85 percent of all back pain.

According to the Mayo Clinic, back pain is often caused by nerve pinching, spinal cord interference, and firing of pain receptors in and around the spine due to spinal malfunction or disorder.

Muscles around the spine can be a secondary source of back pain. Spinal disorders often trigger surrounding muscles into spasm and to stop spinal motion in order to protect the spine from further injury. Such spasms can be highly painful.

Back pain can be disabling. Fear will only make it worse. Bed rest or sitting on the couch for prolonged periods often exaggerates the pain. Moderate and continuous motion and activities, such as:

- Walking,
- Swimming,
- Tai Chi,
- Pilates, and
- Other stretching activities (instead of activities that require bending or twisting of the spine, such as gardening, cycling and golfing)

are the best friends to back pain sufferers, especially acute back pain sufferers.

As long as it doesn't worsen the pain, moderate activities can help improve blood circulation to the muscles, nutrition supply to the discs and accelerate rehabilitation.

They also help reduce or prevent muscle spasms as a secondary pain that, in term of intensity, could often surpass the primary pain.

This may be one of the reasons why physiotherapy and massage therapy have been proven highly effective in back pain management. However, without addressing the cause of primary back pain, the secondary pain may return and the back pain may continue dragging on to become a chronic condition. Often chiropractic care has been proven to be effective in relieving back pain especially the primary pain.

3

11 Secret Causes For Your Continued Suffering

Each year, back pain is almost as common as colds and flu. In fact, back pain is the leading cause for doctor visits, second only to cold and flu. Why then is back pain so pervasive? The problem is the result of the combined effect of many reasons, instead of one single reason. The following is a list of some key issues that have caused the dilemma. Among all these issues, one of the main reasons may be the lack of competence of the mainstream medical care professionals, and the shortcomings in public education, early detection and treatment of the various spinal health issues in their infancy.

1.   Most people take their back and spine for granted due to confusion or lack of motivation. There is no reason to blame ourselves for our shortcomings in taking care of our spine. However, there is also no reason to blame the world for our own back pain. The truth is that if we are motivated to take care of our spine and back as much as we do for our teeth, if we know how to take care of them, and if we do indeed take care of them, most back pain can be

avoided.

2.   Most people do not use their body properly at work or in their daily activities. We may not have kept a heavy object close to our body, or may have used our back instead of our legs to lift it. We may have not stretched our back before intensive exercise. We may have not rotated our head and neck during prolonged driving. You may have shoveled snow with your back bent forward in a "C" shape for a long time. You may not have taken sufficient breaks. Snow removal, whether with a shovel or a snow blower, is strenuous work. You need to take a break of three to five minutes for every 15 to 20-minutes of snow removal work. Otherwise, your posture will be invariably wrong no matter how conscious you were at the beginning. Stress and fatigue naturally lead your body to a poor posture and poor body mechanics for your work, which, over time, often ends in stiffness, pain or fatigue.

3.   You may not have the right sitting foundation and sit still for prolonged periods too often. You may have slouched and sat in a poor posture while working on your computer. You may have not used proper back support to protect your lumbar curvature when sitting in a car seat, an airplane seat, on a couch or in bed. According to the Ontario Workers Safety and Insurance Board (WSIB) in Canada, sitting is a leading cause for lower back injury, second only to heavy weight lifting.

4.   You may have been keeping your head too low. As smart phones and tablets become increasingly pervasive, more and more people are hooked on these types of devices from 2-year-olds to senior citizens. Forward Head Posture (FHP) is one of the leading causes to nagging neck pain. With each inch of forward leaning of our head, the stress and tension in the muscles behind our neck increase by 100 percent. When a person is texting on a smart phone, the head generally protrudes forward 3 to 4 inches, causing the stress and tension in those neck muscles to jump 300 to 400 percent. Figuratively speaking, that person would be carrying 3 to 4 heads on her shoulders while working on her smart phone. Unfortunately, using smart phones and tablets are only two types of the activities we do that lead to Forward Head Posture.

Our head also often leans forward when we:
- Wash our face and brush our teeth,
- Have breakfast,
- Read a newspaper,
- Play with our children or our pets,
- Talk to someone shorter than you,
- Drive a car, if the back of car seat is tilted too far backwards,
- Work on computers,
- Machine a part,
- Work on your craft project,
- Sew a dress,
- Cook a dinner,
- Wash the dishes, or
- Sleep on our back, while using a pillow that's too high for our heads.

Most activities we engage in at work or at home, even when we sleep, our necks are often required or forced to lean forward. Over time, it becomes habitual for us and results in Forward Head Posture which is a clinical condition.

5.   Good spinal alignment and postural stability require good physical strength along with good knowledge, motivation and will. How frequent and how intense your back pain may be upon its return, is often proportional to your physical strength and health. Our spinal vertebrae are held together by a network of ligaments. However, it is the network of muscles surrounding it that ensures the proper alignment. Any weakness or imbalance in these muscles could result in suboptimal alignment of your spine, which often results in future back pain. It is important to know that strong arms do not help reduce or prevent back pains. Neither do strong legs. While working out, you must emphasize the exercises for strengthening and conditioning your back. The most critical stabilizing muscles are directly attached to your spine and are small. However, unlike the big muscles on the arms, legs or in the back, these small stabilizing muscles are very difficult to exercise and strengthen. Most people have weaknesses in these muscles. Due to their small size and shorter range of extension and contraction, you must engage them over a

prolonged period, to improve their condition. Three sets of 10 exercises would not work the same for your back as it does for your arms or legs.

Besides stabilizing muscles, one must also exercise and strengthen the core muscles as a whole. Core muscles are various groups of muscles surrounding your trunk and pelvis. They are the key to proper alignment of your spine, and your ability to maintain a healthy posture, and your ability to protect your back and spine in your daily activities. Core muscles are the foundation of your core stability that is, in turn, the foundation of your posture.

6. Women that wear high heels may notice wearing high heels causes the pelvis to rotate forward, increasing the curvature of the back – known as the lumbar lordosis -- which increases the downward slipping or shearing force placed on the lower lumber discs, which, over time, often leads to back pain, or even a slipped disc. It also increases the wear and tear of the posterior vertebral joints. Increased lumbar lordosis also forces the upper body to compensate by bending the thoracic (upper back) backward and the cervical (neck) spine forward, which, over time, could lead to flat upper back, forward head posture and neck pain. High heels may be in fashion, but can compromise a woman's beauty from the side, because of the visible forward head posture it creates. If a woman is aware of this condition caused by her high heels, she may consciously keep her head up and try to reduce the forward leaning of her head. This forces her pelvis to rotate forward even more and further worsens the biomechanics of her pelvis and lower back which further increases the downward slipping force on the discs in her lower back and the risk of injury and damage to her lower spinal discs and joints.

7. Obesity not only increases the load on the vertebrae and discs from body weight, but also changes the body's structure, balance and spinal biomechanics. Similar to wearing high heels, increased belly mass and weight forces the lumbar spine to bend backward, which increases lumbar lordosis and the shearing forces placed on the lower lumbar discs, which, in turn, increases the risk of damage and misalignment of the lower lumbar vertebrae. As in the case of high heels, increased lumbar lordosis also forces the upper body to compensate by bending the thoracic spine forward, which

over time could lead to forward head posture and neck pain.

8.   Overloading your body by carrying too much weight. This happens most often to school children. Their tender and growing bodies often have to carry school bags weighing as much as half of their body weight. Heavy back packs not only put an enormous load on a child's tender spine but also changes the biomechanics due to asymmetrical loading on the front and back sides of a child's body (the sagittal plane). It forces a child's upper body and head to lean forward in order to balance the load on the back. It also forces their shoulders to roll forward in order to prevent the heavy pack from slipping down.

9.   Emotional stress can cause back pain. Studies have clearly linked emotional stress with back pain. Researchers were even able to predict back pain reoccurrence through analysis of back pain sufferer's emotional stress. Such stress from one's own family is amongst the highest risk factors for back pain.

10.   Inadequate nutrition can harm your back. This is the flipside of the importance of good nutrition. Proper nutrition can help reduce back pain, especially in helping reduce the frequency and intensity of recurring back pain. Poor nutrition could do the reverse, especially, in the case of the back pain associated with inflammation.

11.   Treating the symptoms instead of the causes may make your back angry. You may feel that any sixth grader would understand that the key is to treat the cause if a sustainable result is desired. However, you may be surprised about how often back pain sufferers are simply sent home with a pain killer or a cold pack without a proper effort to diagnose the cause. As discussed before, back pain is only an alarm signal. Treating back pain without treating the cause is like covering up the fire alarm of a burning house. Stopping the alarm doesn't stop the fire. And it is the fire that will destroy the house. Some causes may not be easy to diagnose. However,, you have to identify and treat the cause to prevent the pain from worsening or repeating.

4

5 Categories of Secret Causes Of Your Back Pain

Back pain can be caused by a wide range of conditions. It can be caused by a strain to or a damage of muscles. This type of back pain can be dull or sharp and may get worse with sitting, standing, walking, or other movement. Lying down often helps. In most cases, muscle pain does not extend down your leg. If your back pain shoots down into your leg or legs or even your foot or feet, then there are most likely additional causes for your pain, such as a herniated disc.

Back pain can be caused by inflammation of the muscle, tendons or ligaments. This type of back pain is often constant, both in location and intensity. A hot or cold pack may help. This type of back pain tends to be local and does not vary, travel or radiate to other part or parts of your body.

```
                          ┌──────────────────────┐
                          │  Causes of back pain  │
                          └──────────────────────┘
```

1. in the back	injury
	inflammation
	degeneration
	arthritis
	tension
2. in the pelvis	sacroiliac lesion
	pelvic / ischial-tuberosity obliquity
3. in legs/feet	Pronation of foot
	Supination of foot
	leg length inequality
4. inside the body	inflammation
	stones
	illness
	dehydration, chemical imbalance
	cancers
5. in the mind	emotional stress
	mental stress

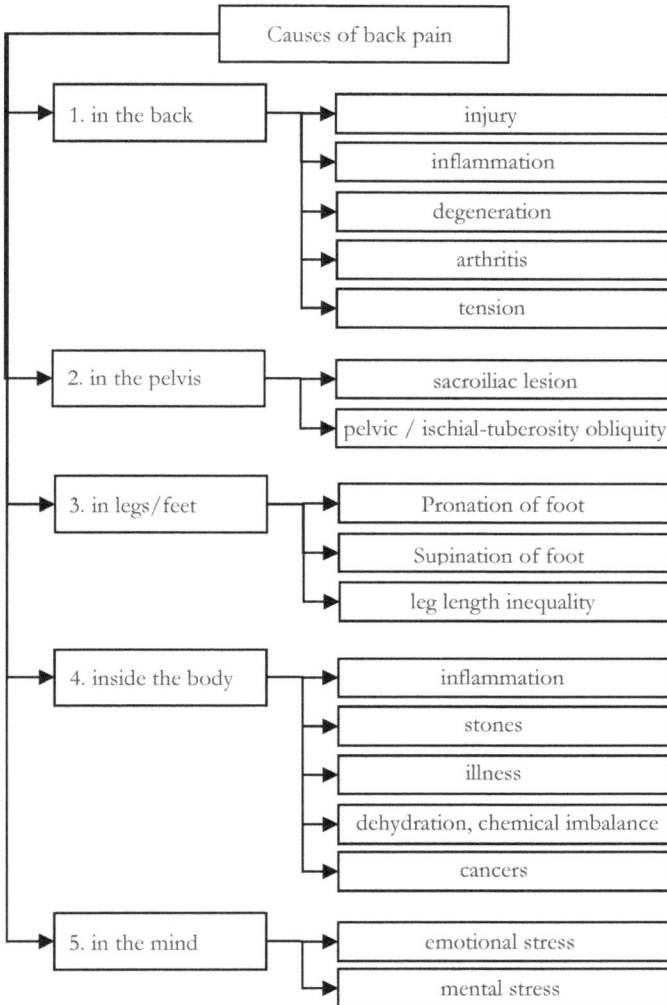

Source: compiled by Patrick Lee

Fig. 1.7

Damaged or degenerated discs can bulge out, pinching the nerve that extends out of the spinal cord between the vertebrae. Back pain caused by a pinched nerve may include numbness, tingling and pain that radiates down the leg, such as sciatica. In severe case of nerve pinching, it can cause problems with controlling your bowels or bladder.

In severe disc dysfunction, the disc may shear and cause adjacent vertebrae to misalign from each other, which, in turn, pinches the related nerves and leads to back pain.

Back pain can also be caused by degeneration, deformation, inflammation or damage of the bony vertebrae,. Degenerated spinal vertebrae can lead to deformation of the vertebrae, which, in turn, often leads to a pinched nerve. Many people experience spinal stenosis in which the nerve canal in the spine narrows and leads to pressure on the nerves. Inflammation can lead to arthritis causing pain.

Auto accidents often lead to damage to the spine with whiplash as the most frequent complaint. Minor whiplash may result in muscle damage, while severe whiplash may result in damage to the vertebrae in the neck.

While a hard to bear back pain is often the result of direct physical injuries such as trauma, herniated disc or repetitive strains, it can be the result of less direct but more severe problems such as cancer. Hence, back pain's underlying health issue require immediate medical attention, especially if the pain is accompanied by such symptoms as unexplained weight loss or fever.

The so called non-specific back pain often involves damage to soft spinal tissues, such as muscles, ligaments, tendons and fascia (the connective tissue fibers underneath the skin, around our muscles, bones, nerves, blood vessels and internal organs). This is often caused by trauma, such as a sudden pull or tear in a sports or auto accident, or caused by repetitive strains present in many professions that involve heavy weight lifting, bending of the back or prolonged sitting.

You may think you were resting when you sat down. Wrong! You are resting your legs and feet only. In most situations, you are making your back work harder when you sit.

Our body is not built for sitting. Most seats and chairs are not designed to support our back. You or those you know may have an expensive chair at work, but still end up with stiffness, fatigue, aches or pains in the back after a few hours of sitting in front of a computer. That is your body's way of telling you that your back is not properly supported. Sitting without a proper foundation to the buttocks or without proper support to the back will start to damage your back in as little as 20-minutes.

Back pains fall into two categories:

1. The acute causes and;
2. The chronic causes.

Acute causes are those that take place suddenly, without forewarning, such as an accident. The chronic causes are those that build themselves up gradually often over the years, even decades, such as osteoarthritis, and then like the last straw on a camel's back, they result in noticeable pain.

However, acuteness of a back pain's cause may not be directly linked to the acuteness of a back pain. Chronic cause may lead to an acute pain, while an acute cause may be linked to a chronic pain.

1. Causes of Pain In Your Back

a. Sprains and Strains

A sprain is a sudden microscopic stretch to the ligaments, while a strain is a sudden microscopic stretch to the muscles or tendons. In the spine, these two conditions are closely associated with each other. One would rarely happen without the other.

Such stretches are often less than 1 mm long. However, to the muscles and the ligaments that are not prepared, it often leads to microscopic tears to the soft tissue cells and their associated microscopic blood vessels, causing local bleeding, or bruising, and pain caused by irritation of the nerve endings in the area. To prevent further tear damage, affected and surrounding tissues often automatically start to contract and lead to spasms that can also be painful. This happens when the content of the torn tissue and blood cells leak out and irritate the surrounding muscle cells that react by contracting.

While muscles and ligaments are soft and flexible in general, in the milliseconds when they are suddenly and unexpectedly stretched, they behave more like a hard and fragile material such as porcelain due to lack of reaction time, and break without much stretching deformation.

You may have experienced this when you heard a sharp and loud sound behind you and quickly turned your head to see what happened, or when you tried to quickly lift up a heavy bin from the ground without preparing your back for it. In both actions, your sudden movements may have caused muscle spasms and pain in your lower back, from the unexpected stretching of the muscles and ligaments.

This is why it is critical to stretch your body before intense exercises. Stretch your back before you pick up that garbage bag, that case of beer or lift a heavy suitcase.

Rotate your head and neck during long office sitting hours, or on long car rides especially if you are the driver. Otherwise your head will be fixed in one position and direction for a long time and be highly prone to stretch pain when you suddenly need to turn your head to observe traffic behind you or answer your phone.

As we age, the time the muscles need to react to sudden stretches increases. Thus the risk from such muscle pain increases with an individual's age. Therefore, proper movement and stretching before intensive exercise or during a prolonged period of sitting or standing in the same unchanged posture becomes increasingly important with our age.

On the other hand, it is nature's self-protective mechanism, in which our body starts to slow down and engage in less sudden twists, turns, and bending. If an older person did as many sudden twists, turns, and bending as teenagers did, he or she would be afflicted by stretch pains nonstop.

Ligament sprain and muscle strain-caused pains often can't be detected by X-ray, CT or MRI scans because most such injuries don't cause visible tissue deformation on these medical imaging devices.

They can be sharp and intense at times, however, they are relatively harmless to your health, and will generally heal within a few weeks. You don't need to trouble a healthcare professional, because nothing can help it heal, but your own body, which needs time. Give it a few weeks; you will become better in most situations.

In case the cause of your back pain is well understood and is being taken care of, you may choose to take some pain killers or use cold or hot packs to take the edge off the pain.

Whatever you do, remain active. Keep motion in your body by walking, swimming, and by doing house chores that do not require much bending and twisting of your spine. Motion is the best friend of your back when back pain hits. Do not lie down beyond your required normal sleep, and do not sit still or stand still for prolonged periods.

The sharpness and intensity of your back pain is not necessarily proportional to the severity of the underlying injury or problem in your back, nor is it proportional to the duration that the pain and/or its underlying cause need to dissipate or to heal. Don't be intimidated by your back pain. Don't ignore light pains in your back, but also don't fear sharp and intense ones. Deal with them cautiously. Find the cause or causes before using any pain killers, unless the pain itself is killing you.

b. Facet Joint Irritation

On the back of the vertebral bones are smaller bony projections that are linked with the next vertebral bone via two pairs of bony facets and associated tissue called synovium. The bony facets and synovium allow the spine to twist and bend as desired, and also limit the range of motion to protect the spinal cord. However, the facets can be irritated and cause pain. The pain can be severe, but only with certain movement that compresses or stretches the affected facet.

Such irritation mostly happens in the most mobile sections of the spine, such as the lower back and the neck, because the facet joints are highly prone to wear and tear, and degeneration. If one lives long enough, the facet joints will be worn and torn to the degree such irritation will occur, because it is a natural process of aging.

It could be caused by abnormal wear and tear or spinal degeneration, in which case the cartilage may be worn out and lead to direct bone contact between the adjacent vertebral bones. The vertebral bones react to such direct contact by producing additional bone mass leading to osteoarthritis and facet inflammation that cause significant pain when bodily motion requires the involvement of the affected facet joint. The inflammation causes the surrounding muscles to go into spasms in an automatic natural self-protection of the facet joint.

Such muscle spasms not only become a secondary source of severe pain, but also causes spinal lesion. Treatment of such pain requires relaxation of affected muscles instead of realignment of the affected vertebrae. However, realignment of affected vertebral may help reduce facet joint irritation, thus the secondary pain.

c. Herniated Disc

Some statistics indicate that herniated discs are responsible for only a small portion of all lower back pain.

The disc has a gel like core called a nucleus surrounded by two layers of annulus. Under extreme pressure or when the annulus is weakened, the gel like nucleus may force the annulus to deform to such an extent, it forces the surrounding ligament outward to touch upon the spinal cord or the nerve roots. In extreme cases, the nucleus may even break through the annulus and directly force the surrounding ligament outward, even breaking through the ligament wall to press against the spinal cord or the nerve's roots.

Herniated discs most often occur in the lower back. Depending on the location of the disc, it often causes pain that shoots down the leg along the pathway of the affected nerve exiting the spine. This condition is often thought to be a pinched nerve.

The nerves exiting the second, third, and fourth lumbar vertebral joints (often labeled by medical professionals as L2, L3 and L4), these joints join together to form the femoral nerves, that control everything of the front thigh. The nerves exiting the fourth, fifth, and first three sacrum vertebral joints form the sciatic nerve that is the largest nerve in human body and controls everything in the back, the thigh, the legs, and the feet. Since most herniated discs occur in the L4, L5, or L5 S1 vertebrae joints, it is most often associated with sciatica.

Severe herniated discs often require surgical intervention, while mild to medium herniated discs can be taken care of by less invasive manual treatment, such as chiropractic or osteopath care.

d. Compression Fractures

Aging and poor health can cause compression fractures of the vertebral body. Osteoporosis is the most common cause of this situation. When this happens, you may feel a sudden and sharp pain around the location where the facture took place. The pain may radiate around your rib cage, if it happens in your mid back. Alternatively, the pain may radiate around your pelvis or down your leg, if the fracture took place in the lower back.

It is worthwhile to note that you may want to stay away from any manual treatments such as chiropractic, osteopath, physiotherapy, massage therapy and so on, because these therapies are not able to treat fractured vertebrae.

The good news is that a compression fracture often heals itself within several weeks without requiring any special treatment. In such a situation, having an X-ray, a CT or an MRI scan to confirm the condition is often the best treatment. Then relax, and let your body heal itself.

The bad news is that the shape of your vertebral body and your spinal curvature may suffer permanent deformation. Such deformation may lead to a change of biomechanics of your spine, such as hunched back (hyperkyphosis), scoliosis, or an increase on the wear and tear of your spinal joints. This may lead to more back and joint stress and cause unexpected pain down the road.

e. Spinal Degeneration

Spinal degeneration affects not only the vertebral bodies and facet joints, but also spinal discs. Degeneration of facet joints often leads to osteoarthritis.

Degeneration of discs often leads to thinned discs, which on one hand causes the exit canal of the nerves to narrow, which may interfere with the exiting nerve roots and cause pain. On the other hand, it also causes adjacent vertebral bodies to touch and rub against each other, which contributes to the degeneration of the vertebral bodies.

The degeneration of vertebral body leads to growth of the bony spurs around the vertebrae. This condition is referred to as spondylosis. And the bony spurs are called osteophytes. As the bony spurs or osteophytes grow bigger, they may begin to protrude into the central nerve canal, a condition called stenosis which essentially narrows the spinal canal and eventually interferes with the spinal cord and causes pain.

f. Disc Displacement

Disc Displacement (also known as disc slippage) is the forward or backward displacement of vertebra, relative to the one underneath it. It occurs when a disc has fallen out of its alignment in the spine.

Most Disc Displacements happen between the fifth lumbar vertebra and the first sacrum vertebra (i.e., at the L5/S1 joint), due to an especially disadvantaged biomechanical condition of the spinal disc (the greatest downward slope of the disc) there. Such Disc Displacement is also referred as spondylolisthesis.

The discs in the lower lumbar area become increasingly sloped downward. The lower a disc is located in the spine, the more sloped it is, and the more the body weight and the external load transform into a downward shearing force, putting stress on the disc.

And the disc between L5 and S1 has the most pronounced slope among all discs -- so it bears the highest level of stress, and thus the highest risk to lead to the displacement of adjacent vertebrae.

Spondylolisthesis is often the result of the spinal degeneration. When spinal discs degenerate, they become less and less capable of resisting the shearing forces placed on them by body weight and the loads we carry. This mostly happens in the lumbar region, especially at locations of L5/S1 and L4/L5 because the shearing force is at its highest on these discs due to the fact that the downward sloping angles of the discs is at its steepest, and the fact that the body weight and external load that need to be supported by the spinal discs are at their highest too.

When the disc is no longer capable of holding the body's weight and the load placed on it, it slips forward and downward causing spondylolisthesis to occur and the spinal canal to narrow and may begin to jam the spinal nerves.

Backward displacement is referred to as retrolisthesis which is very rare, and does not commonly happen at L5/S1. It is also not often the result of spinal degeneration. Rather, it is frequently caused by spinal trauma or abnormal spine curvature.

Both forward and backward Disc Displacement are a serious conditions. Patients often need to take on highly invasive treatments, such as surgery.

It is helpful to realize that non-invasive treatments such as chiropractic, osteopath, physiotherapy, massage therapy are usually not effective in treating such conditions, because they usually are not able to restore a displaced disc.

g. Disc Tear

A disc tear is often the result of spinal degeneration too. As we age, the layers of the disc wall (annulus) gradually weakens. Microscopic tears may emerge in the belt like wall layers of the disc. A biochemical called Cytokines may leak through the tear from the jelly centre (nucleus) of the disc to reach the pain sensing outer one third of layers of disc wall to cause pain and cause an inflammation in the outer disc wall that reinforces the pain. Leakage of the nucleus also decreases the capacity of evenly distributing the spinal pressure over the surface of the disc.

As a result, the pressure distribution shifts from the entire disc surface to concentrate on the posterior part of the disc or the annulus. Such dramatically increased pressure on the pain-sensitive outer annulus on the back of the disc, together with the inflammation caused by the Cytokines, can create severe pain in the spinal disc – often referred to as discogenic pain. Interestingly, some people may suffer a disc tear but not any pain. Explanation to this situation is yet to be found.

h. Poor Posture

Typical poor posture includes a slouched back when sitting, a forward head posture, a hunched back, and an anterior pelvic tilt that often happens when wearing high heels, during pregnancy or when obesity is present.

Poor posture weakens the spinal ligament and fatigues back muscles, both of which increases the risk of herniated or slipped discs. Poor posture also leads to:

- Increased tension,
- Increased asymmetry
- Reduced blood circulation,
- Increased waste
- Increased repetitive strains and
- Increased risk of repetitive strain injury in the associated back muscles.

Poor posture may worsen the biomechanics of the spine. Poor posture also causes repetitive injuries to associated back muscles and ligaments.

Poor posture can damage the spine and afflict back pain in many ways. For example, a disc hernia is common with computer workers, that tend to slouch most of the time they sit. Neck pain and upper back pain is pervasive among office workers. Back pain is pervasive amongst truck drivers, taxi drivers, pilots, and public transit drivers.

Based on their causes, poor posture can be generally divided into three main categories:

1. **Conditional Poor Posture**: Such poor postures are generally forced by an external environment, such as in the case of sitting in a car on a seat that provides little or no support to the back. This forces the back into a forward facing "C" curve. Or in the case of working in a confined environment, such as in a mine, where workers are forced to lay low, by

bending their backs. Other examples where the external environment or conditions may bring about a Conditional Poor Posture include, working in front of a computer, machining a part, texting on a smart phone, ironing a shirt, cooking a meal, or planting flowers.

To reduce or prevent Conditional Poor Posture, it is almost always required to modify the environment or condition surrounding you, such as applying a suitable back support when you sit in a car or airplane seat, or properly realign your seat, desk and computer monitor.

2. **Habitual Poor Posture**: Such poor postures generally occur due to one's individual habits. For example, many people slouch when working in front of a computer. In the case that many people walk or stand with their heads forward protruded, instead of keeping them up right and properly aligned with their spine. Alternatively, some people walk or stand, with their chest closed and their shoulders rolling forward, instead of keeping them open and straight. Or in the case that many people sleep on their side, with their bodies curled up like a shrimp. You may say: "Oh, please! Could you just relax?! You are even talking about my sleep. I just want to have a comfortable sleep. The shrimp-like posture in sleep doesn't cause any stress or tension in any muscles." You are right that a poor posture during sleep generally creates little or no stress to any muscles, tendons or ligaments. However they will cause an asymmetrical plastic stretch which can lead to muscular imbalances during the day. What may be more damaging is the effect of the curling up of your body on the neurological patterning of your muscles, tendons, ligaments and joints which are the keys for your life. Eight-hours of sleep is one-third of your day. It is a very long time as far as the posture is concerned. You rarely maintain your body in one posture more than four-hours, let alone eight-hours, unless your body is forced by a living or working condition, such as taking a long flight on an airplane.
    It is very difficult for you to do anything during the day to neutralize the slouching effect from your sleep, because the

neurological patterning effect is largely proportional to time, and you simply don't have enough time to combat the slouching effects of your sleep during the day, assuming that you have a normal active life.

To reduce or prevent Habitual Poor Posture, it is almost always required to re-educate the mind. Too many therapies or devices have been focused on helping strengthen the muscles. For example, many doctors and therapists advise their patients with Forward Head Posture repeatedly press their head backwards against an elastic band pulled forward by two hands, for resistance training for the neck muscles. Such treatments assume that strengthened muscles would serve to keep the body straight. However, the reality is that the muscles are almost always strong enough to keep the body straight. It is the mind that subconsciously or even consciously tells the muscles to stop doing their jobs before they pull the body into a straight posture. The causes to many spinal problems are neuromechanical in nature, as opposed to be purely biomechanical in nature.

3. **Anatomical/Pathological Poor Posture**: Such poor postures are generally caused by some illnesses, injuries or abnormalities, such as a compressive fracture of the spine or scoliosis. A compressive fracture of the spine causes your spine to overtly curve forward no matter what you do – regardless of how strong your awareness and desire is for a good posture, how perfect your working or living environment may be, or how much effort you make to combat it.
Or in the case of a scoliosis that may have come from birth and forces your spine to curve abnormally.
Or in the case that you have a temporary stomach ache that forces you to bend your back forward to feel better.

To reduce or prevent Anatomical/Pathological Poor Posture, invasive treatment is often required, unfortunately.

What could you do to combat these three categories of slouches?

For conditional slouches, you need to examine and improve your environment. For example, if you are a taxi driver, a truck driver, a pilot or just someone who spends long hours traveling in vehicles or on airplanes, you could add a well-designed back support to your seat to provide the back support needed and prevent your lumbar curvature from being flattened or reversed.

"Oh, I am driving a premium automobile and have a great seat. So I don't need a back support," you may think.

You may be right if you are driving an ultra-high-end luxury car. However the seat design of an average Mercedes, BMW, Audi, or Jaguar simply doesn't provide proper back support. Next time you sit in such a luxury automobile, pay attention to how your lumbar curvature compares with the one you have when you stand tall and straight. You will realize that your lumbar lordosis has been compromised, even reversed!

The same problem exists with airplane seats, even the first class seats. If those luxury automobile and airplane seats can't provide adequate support to the back, imagine the non-luxury cars and airplane seats most of us use daily. If you don't have a properly designed back support in your car or that you take with you while flying, you are likely damaging your back each time you travel.

What could you do if you have a habitual slouch? You need to examine and improve your sitting habits. Changing your habits may be easier said than done, because, in most cases, poor habits occur subconsciously -- when you are not aware of it.

What you need to do is to retrain your muscles, tendons, ligaments, joints and brain to re-establish your healthy neurological pattern, to one of good posture.

However, it is also not that difficult to achieve good and healthy habits. Clear understanding of the phenomena, its cause, and what you need to do is already a great first step. Next, need to learn what good postures are in various situations, such as standing, sitting, walking and sleeping.

You can also look into the many exercises, therapies, and products that can help you re-establish your healthy posture, such as:

- Yoga
- The Alexander technique
- Pilates exercises
- Sleeping on your back (with a thin pillow that has a firm neck

support) instead of on your side
- Applying a dynamic stability seat when you sit

What could you do if you have an anatomical or pathological slouch? You need to see a spine specialist to resolve the underlying cause.

However, not every cause for an anatomical or a pathological slouch needs to be resolved, such as compressive fractures. The spine often heals itself within a number of weeks, and often doesn't experience any pain long after words.

Certainly the significant forward protrusion of the head and shoulder caused by compressive fractures greatly increases the stress and tension in the related back muscles, tendons and ligaments, and leads to greatly increased wear and tear of the spine.

Unfortunately, the solution to deal with a compressive fracture is often an invasive surgery which has risks and negative side effects.

Is it worth the risk to go through an invasive procedure to deal with potential musculoskeletal problems down the road?

To most, the answer may be negative. However, such debates and decisions are highly sensitive on a case-by-case basis. No general answer can be provided. If you face such a dilemma, you must seek consultation by a qualified spine specialist.

i.   Impaired Function of Spinal Joint

Like when our stomach suffers an indigestion and needs the puncture of the acupuncture needle,   or a computer freezes and needs a reboot, our spine may experience various degrees of impaired function and need a relief. Some of these may result in back pain and less optimal function of the body and organs. Such Impaired Function is often referred to as Subluxation within Chiropractic care.

According to World Health Organization, chiropractic subluxation is: "a lesion or dysfunction in a joint or motion segment in which alignment, movement integrity and/or physiological function are altered, although contact between joint surfaces remains intact. It is essentially a functional entity, which may influence biomechanical and neural integrity."

This definition also indicates that a lesion or a dysfunction of the spinal joint could result in more than just back pain, when such a lesion affects the nerve roots which, according to the outside-in (somatoviscero) nature of the body, can affect the function of associated body parts or organ either positively or negatively.

Although medical professionals of various disciplines argue about the validity of the chiropractic subluxation concept, this concept and its associated treatments have made chiropractic care the care of choice with the highest satisfaction ranking among all treatments for back pain, as rated by a Consumer Report survey of 14,000 back pain sufferers in 2013. See details below in this book.

Do you want to be right, or do you want to be pain free?

j. Repetitive Strain Injury

Repetitive strain injury affects more than the hands, wrists, and elbows. It can cause debilitating injuries to your back too. Neck, shoulders, and upper back are among the most common areas affected by repetitive strain injury. Repetitive symptoms may include pain, aching, tenderness, stiffness, and numbness.

In the initial stage, symptoms may only occur when you are doing a particular repetitive action, and improve when you have finished the action. If nothing is done to take care of the situation, the condition may worsen and enter the second stage in which the affected area may swell. If the condition continues worsening and enters the third stage, your injury may become chronic.

Overuse, poor posture, and poor body mechanics are the key causes of repetitive strain injury.

k. Muscular Tension

Muscle tension is a condition in which muscles remain semi-contracted for an extended period. Muscle tension is typically caused by:

- Physiological stress,
- Inflammation or damage,
- Poor posture,
- And conditions, such as scoliosis, an uneven pelvis, or uneven legs.

Muscular tension can cause back pain if it happens in the back.

Stress may cause the nervous system to constrict blood vessels and reduce blood flow to the soft tissues, including muscles, tendons, and nerves. This process causes oxygen starvation and buildup of biochemical waste in the muscles, which in turn, results in muscle tension, spasms, and pain. Such stress may be physical, mental or emotional. Many stressors may be in chemical forms too, from poor nutrition, to drugs, and environmental pollution.

Inflammation and damage of joints and soft tissues may trigger the body's self-protective mechanism, which causes the surrounding muscles to tense and prevent further motion in the affected area. Such a process is also accompanied by oxygen starvation and a buildup of biochemical waste in the affected muscles, which in turn, results in stiffness and pain.

Poor posture often causes muscles to behave asymmetrically, some contracting while others stretching, for prolonged periods. This leads to extra stress and tension in the back muscles, tendons and ligaments.

Conditions, such as scoliosis, uneven pelvis or uneven legs, may turn the stress and tension that occurs due to poor posture, into a semi-permanent state, and cause exaggerated pain.

Muscle tension can often be successfully treated by:

- Gentle therapeutic exercises,
- Massage,
- Acupuncture,
- Acupressure,
- Laser,
- Infrared,
- Heat,
- And water therapy.

1. Hyper Mobility

Many of us have seen someone that appears to be double-jointed, such as bending their thumbs backwards to their wrists, stretching their fingers further than normal, bending their knee backwards – maybe they can even cross their legs behind their head or perform other amazing feats that a contortionist would do for an audience.

These individuals have hyper mobility in the parts of their body they can stretch further than normal.

Although it may be amazing to watch someone stretch and bend further than normal, people with hyper mobility may be more prone to sprains, strains and pains in their joints, spine and back.

Hyper mobility of the joints is mainly caused by ligament laxity (or "loose ligaments") and disc degeneration.

Ligament laxity may be the result of aging, genetics, or improper use of the body, of which poor posture plays a big part. Disc degeneration leads to thinner discs, which in turn leads to looser ligaments. Imagine a person wearing his normal clothes after losing half of his body weight. The clothes would fit loosely on the body. Think of the clothes as your ligaments, and degenerated discs as the body that lost half of its weight. The ligaments would become loose just as the clothes did in our example.

Ligament laxity may be especially harmful to the spin by leading to vertebral segmental movement out of sync with the collective motion patterns of the spine. Hypermobility may present as increased, uncontrolled and undesirable movements compared to what is expected. As a result, the joints may become more susceptible to injury and the muscles surrounding the joints may have to work harder to stabilize the affected joints. Prolonged overwork may lead to decrease of the blood supply and increase of the build-up of lactic acid causing pain. Such prolonged overwork may also lead to repetitive strain injury to the muscles and associated pain.

Hypermobility in the spine (segmental hypermobility) may also lead to disc degeneration, and later it could even progress to spinal instability (segmental instability) which may then lead to nerve compression in the spine and severe pain in the back and other parts of the body.

m. Arthritis

There are a number of types of arthritis that can affect the back. The most common is osteoarthritis. The second most common type of arthritis affecting the back is rheumatoid arthritis, while the third most common is psoriatic arthritis. Viral and bacterial infections, and their related arthritis (such as septic arthritis) rarely affect spinal joints.

Osteoarthritis is mostly caused by aging, injury, overuse, or poor spinal care that cause premature spinal degeneration. Osteoarthritis can cause pain in most parts of the spine, however, mostly in the lower back or the neck where the spine is most prone to wear, tear, and degeneration.

Rheumatoid arthritis is caused by an autoimmune disorder. When your immune system, which defends your body against disease, starts thinking healthy cells as foreign, and begins attacking these healthy cells, you have an autoimmune disorder. An autoimmune disease can affect many different types of body tissues and parts of the body.

It can also affect joints in the back, but while mainly in the hands. Psoriatic arthritis is an autoimmune disorder and can cause pain in the sacrum.

n. Stenosis

Spinal Stenosis (the narrowing of the spinal canal) is mostly caused by spinal degeneration, but can also be caused by trauma and congenital disorder. Stenosis can cause severe back pain, sciatica, and even paralysis, if it occurs in the neck.

Most commonly, stenosis occurs in the neck and the lumbar spine. While stenosis in the lower back may cause more people to suffer from back pain, the stenosis in the neck is far more dangerous because it may compress upon the spinal cord. Luckily the spinal cord ends at the top section of the lumbar spine, between the first and second lumbar vertebrae. As a result, stenosis in the lower back does not have the risk of compressing the spinal cord. However, it doesn't mean its consequences would not be severe. Stenosis is, unfortunately, a serious condition that normally can't be successfully treated by manual or chemical therapies, and eventually requires surgery.

o. Developmental Bone Problems

Scoliosis (an abnormal sideway curvature in the spine) and Paget's Disease of Bone (an abnormal growth process of bone tissues, especially in the spine) are among the most common developmental bone problems.

Scoliosis is characterized with a sideway "S" curve of the spine. It is categorized in three key groups:

1. Congenital scoliosis starts at birth,
2. Idiopathic scoliosis are those scoliosis whose cause is unknown, and
3. Secondary scoliosis is the result of a primary condition, such as a neuromuscular asymmetry or disorder, physical trauma, spinal degeneration, aging, or Chiari Malformation (structural defects in the cerebellum, the part of the brain that controls balance.)

While congenital and idiopathic scoliosis rarely cause pain, secondary scoliosis does have a considerable risk of causing pain, especially in the case of degenerative scoliosis. Scoliosis affects the spine and causes back pain in many ways, most commonly through muscle tension and premature spinal degeneration to form a vicious circle.

Paget's Disease of the Bone is a chronic disorder of excessive breakdown and formation of bone that result in abnormal shape and size of bones and disorganized bone alignment. It weakens the affected bones, causes pain, fractures, and arthritis in the joints around the affected bones. Paget's Disease of Bone is typically localized to only a few bones in the lower lumbar spine, the pelvis, and the femur (thigh bone).

Developmental Bone Problems often result in abnormal spinal alignment and worsened biomechanical condition for the vertebrae and discs, which in term may lead to abnormal muscle stress and tension, reduced range of motion, premature spinal degeneration, increased risk of injury and pain.

p. Piriformis Syndrome

Piriformis syndrome is a condition where the sciatic nerve is compressed or otherwise irritated by the piriformis muscle. The piriformis muscle is a pair of muscles that run over the sciatic nerves, rotate around the hips outward, and help keep the body stable and upright when moving around.

In 15 percent of the population, the sciatic nerves actually run directly through the piriformis muscles. The nerve compression or irritation happens when the piriformis muscles tighten or spasm due to strain or overuse.

Piriformis syndrome can cause pain, tingling, and numbness in the buttocks and along the path of the sciatic nerve down into the legs.

2. Causes of Back Pain In Your Pelvis

If we say that the spine is foundation to the back, then the pelvis is the foundation of the spine. Anything that goes wrong with the pelvis will often affect the function and the wellness of the spine, and hence the back. Ligament injury can cause back pain. Unevenness of the structure of the position of the pelvis can cause problems in the spine and create back pain too.

a. Sacroiliac Ligament Injury or Sacroiliac Lesion

The sacrum is the link that transmits the weight of the upper body including arms, head, and neck to the pelvis, then on to the legs. It is linked with the pelvis with tough and strong ligaments only, without any muscle. The weight of the upper body and any load our body lifts or carries has a tendency to push the sacrum downwards relative to the pelvis.

When the sacroiliac ligaments are weakened or the upper body weight or load it carries is too high, the ligaments may become injured and allow microscopic movements between the sacrum and the ilium - its socket on the pelvis. This injury and the micro movement of the sacrum can cause severe lower back pain that also shoots down the legs.

Sacroiliac ligament injury happens with no involvement of any muscle because the sacrum is connected with the ilium through the ligaments only. Such injuries often lead to a lesion or dislocation of the sacrum relative to the ilium. Such dislocation can be severe, however, in most cases, they are minor. Such injuries and lesions can be caused by trauma, such as slips, falls, car accidents, and sports activities.

They can also be caused by poor posture. Poor posture affects the sacrum as a continuously progressing micro stretch to the ligaments. Slouching in a chair for hours at a time can lead to the ligaments being stretched so much that the sacrum starts to slip relative to the ilium.

The sacroiliac lesion can also be brought on by pregnancy. A woman's body releases a hormone to relax the ligaments in preparation for delivery. Such ligament relaxation may lead to hypermobility in the sacroiliac and other joints. With increased body weight, such hypermobility of the sacroiliac joints may lead to spinal lesion and back pain.

Sacroiliac ligament injuries and lesions can also be caused by daily activities, such as bending, twisting, and lifting. The stiffer the flexible portion of the back, especially the lower back, the higher the risk of sacroiliac ligament injury. That is because the flexible portion of the back or spine is designed to take the load of the bending and twisting motions of the back. The higher the body weight or the heavier the object the body lifts or carries, the higher the risk of sacroiliac ligament injury.

Obesity doesn't only affect one's appearance, it affects one's bodily structure and back health. And the way in which obesity affects one's back health is not limited to the merely increased body weight that sacroiliac ligaments have to bear. It also damages the back by changing the biomechanics of the shearing forces on the spinal discs especially on the discs in the lower back. More on this later.

b. Ischial Tuberosity Obliquity

The sitting bones (ischial tuberosities) may sometimes be uneven in length. If the pelvis were a stool, and the sitting bones were its legs, the stool would tilt if the legs were uneven in length. When sitting bones are uneven in length, the pelvis will tilt sideways or laterally when a person sits down. If the spine is planted in the pelvis like a tall building in a foundation, the spine will tilt when the pelvis is not leveled.

To maintain the balance of the upper body, the spine will be forced to compensate this tilt by bending towards the opposite direction. This not only increases the stress and tension in the back muscles and ligaments, but also may lead to soft tissue imbalances, even scoliosis, over time.

Ischial tuberosity obliquity affects different people differently. For a person who is constantly on their feet, it may not cause many problems. However, for a person who frequently sits for long periods of time, such as office workers, taxi or truck drivers, pilots, or wheelchair users, ischial tuberosity obliquity may bring significant challenges to the back and the spine. As our society becomes increasingly sedentary, spinal problems and back pains caused by ischial tuberosity obliquity have become more prevalent.

Typical consequences may include sore back, back stiffness, back pains, scoliosis, premature spinal degeneration, herniated discs, and headaches.

c. Pelvic Obliquity

The tilt of the pelvis may not only be caused by ischial tuberosity obliquity, but it may also happen due to a number of other issues, such as:

- Piriformis syndrome (also known as "wallet sciatica" or "fat wallet syndrome,") as the condition can stem from sitting on a large wallet,

- Leg length inequality, or
- Hip contracture (a permanent fixation of the hip in a certain position. Movement of hip is difficult and pain may be present when the hip is in motion. It may be caused by trauma, infection, or poliomyelitis).

Unlike ischial tuberosity obliquity and fat wallet syndrome that only causes pelvis obliquity while sitting, leg length inequality and contractures about the hips also cause the pelvic obliquity while standing or walking. As a result leg length inequality and hip contractures can also affect people that are on their feet during most of the day.

Whatever its origin, pelvic obliquity may consequently lead to pressure sores, scoliosis, and hyperlordosis, and may be a silent demon causing you back pain and spinal problems. To fight this demon you must find its origin and cause. Is it in your pelvis, legs, feet, or shoes? Could it be from your standing platform, or your seat?

3. Causes of Back Pain In Your Legs / Feet
If the pelvis is the foundation of the spine, the legs and feet are the foundation of the pelvis. Any unevenness or obliquity in the legs or feet may lead to pelvic obliquity, hence causing trouble in your spine and back.

a. Leg Length Discrepancy
Leg Length Discrepancy is also called Limb Length Discrepancy. Most of us are not perfect creatures. Strictly speaking, our legs are always slightly different in length. According to the American Academy of Orthopedic Surgeons, the normal range of leg length discrepancy is from zero inches, up to three-fifths of an inch. A study involving 600 healthy military recruits showed that 32 percent of them had a one-fifth of an inch to a three-fifths of an inch difference between the lengths of their legs.

Beside natural variances, leg length discrepancy can also be caused by:

- Injuries and diseases, such as injury to a bone in the leg;
- A childhood bone infection,
- Multiple Hereditary Exostoses (HME), a rare condition

where multiple bony spurs or lumps (called "exostoses" or "osteochondromas") develop on the bones of a child, HME can lead to the shortening and bowing of bones, and inequality of limb length, or

- Ollier Disease, a rare disorder which makes the affected extremity shortened (asymmetric dwarfism) and sometimes bowed..

Normally, Leg Length Discrepancy may only begin to become noticeable or start to cause trouble to our health when it exceeds one quarter to one-half of an inch. When the discrepancy is greater than one-half of an inch, you need to seek solutions to mitigate potential risks.

b. Pronation of Foot

A foot may roll inward during normal standing, walking or running, which is referred to as pronation. Pronation of foot can be caused by imbalance of muscles or ligaments in the foot, or malformation of certain bones, or a neurological reaction.

A moderate amount of pronation is natural and required for the proper function of the foot. However, excessive pronation or hyper pronation may cause rotation of the ankle, knee, and leg to cause pelvic obliquity and affect the wellness of the spine and back. It may also lead to damage and injury of the foot, ankle, knee, leg, or hip.

c. Supination of Foot

Supination is the opposite of pronation and refers to the outward rolling of the foot during normal standing, walking, or running. A moderate amount of supination is natural and necessary during some motions, such as the push-off phase of running. However, excessive supination frequently causes pelvic obliquity and may lead to problems in the back and spine.

4. Causes of Back Pain Inside Your Body

The cause of your back pain may be outside of your back. As discussed in the section on viscerosomatic reflex, distress in the inner organs often manifest themselves as pain in phantom back pain. It is important to look into your body for potential causes.

It is critical to separate pain originating from inside the body from those coming from the back itself. While there are many details that need special training to practice, the principle is rather simple and easy.

Here are four simple tips to tell if your back pain is located inside your body:

First, pay attention to any pain or discomfort inside your body. If you have any problem, discomfort or pain with any inner organ, you need to look into the possibility of whether your back pain is actually a manifestation of the problem with your inner organ.

Second, if you have any illness, such as an infection inside your pelvis, or an injury, such as a "kidney punch" from boxing class, and you suffer back pain, you need to carefully look into your internal illness or injury and make sure it is not the primary cause of your back pain. Make sure you take care of the illness or injury with your inner organs and body.

Third, if you have not been diagnosed with any illness of your inner organs, yet you suffer from back pain, then you need to pay attention to any signs that may indicate your body is fighting a problem inside your body. Often, inner organ problems that cause back pain are associated with infection and inflammation. Your body may be hard at work fighting something internally. Signs your body is fighting something inside of you are:

- A higher temperature, even a fever,
- An irregular and/or unsettled stomach,
- Abnormal bowel movements, your urine and stool may appear unusual from normal.

Pay attention to your body's general wellbeing besides the pain in your back.

Fourth, if you have an infection with your inner organs which is healed, however your back pain still continues. If the pain is originating from an infected inner organ, it should stop once the infection is cleared.

If the infection has stopped, but the back pain still continues, there may be three possibilities. First, the pain may be caused by an injured organ which still struggles although its infection is cleared. Second, the pain may be caused by another infected inner organ.

Third, the cause of your back pain is not inside your body, but in your back or in your mind (Not that you dreamed up your pain in your mind. But more on this later).

In a plain langue, if your back pain is accompanied by any pain or discomfort inside your body, your back pain may be associated with or caused by the pain or discomfort inside your body. You need to pay great attention to the problems inside your body, instead of to your back only. You should not use pain killer if you do not pay attention to the issues inside your body. It is good to keep the alarm sound on before its cause is diagnosed and treated.

a. Kidney Problems

Kidney stones and infection often manifest themselves as lower back pain, even as pain in the hips and groin area. Adult kidneys are two fist-sized organs responsible for the detoxification of blood, located at each side of the spine at the lower end of the rib cage, from T12 to L2 level from the vertebral point of view.

Typical signs of kidney infection are:

- Fevers and high temperatures
- Feeling unwell or sick,
- An upset stomach and/or vomiting
- Cloudy, bloody or foul smelling urine, and
- And more frequent urination.

According to Dr. Scott Fishman, chief of the Division of Pain Medicine and professor of Anesthesiology and Pain Medicine at the University of California, Davis: "Pain stemming from a kidney infection typically is in the area of the back where the kidneys lie, located to the sides of the spine, just above the hips."

"Kidney related pain often presents as tenderness in this area. Direct injury or trauma to the back -- over the area where the kidneys are located -- can cause injury to the kidneys themselves," continued Dr. Fishman. "Kidney pain is also quite tricky because it can radiate to many different parts of the body. It is also acute in origin, meaning that it usually has a very rapid onset, and typically does not last any longer than the infection in the kidneys last."

b. Gallbladder Problems

Gallbladder infection, stone, or inflammation can cause pain in the mid-back, the right shoulder, and between the shoulder blades.

Particular conditions include:

- Biliary colic, (the type of pain that occurs when a gallstone transiently obstructs the cystic duct and the gallbladder contracts),
- Cholecystitis, (an inflammation of the gallbladder),
- Gallstones,(small and hard crystals that are formed abnormally in the gallbladder or bile ducts, and can cause severe pain and blockage of the bile duct.)
- Pancreatitis,(inflammation of the pancreas that can lead to severe pain),
- And ascending cholangitis (an infection of the bile duct (cholangitis), usually caused by bacteria ascending from its junction with the first part of the small intestine. Cholangitis can lead to intense pain and be life-threatening).

These conditions cause pain in two ways:

1. Intermittent or a complete blockage of any of the ducts by gallstones;

2. Gallstone sludge and/or inflammation that may accompany irritation or infection of the surrounding tissues, when partial or complete obstruction of ducts causes pressure and ischemia (inadequate blood supply due to a blockage of blood vessels in the area) to develop in the adjacent tissues.

And such pains can manifest themselves in the back to be perceived as back pain. You want to seek immediate care if the following signs and symptoms of a serious gallstone complication develop:

- Abdominal pain so severe that you can't find a comfortable position.

- Yellowing of your skin and the whites of your eyes.

- High fever with chills.

Women are more likely than men to suffer from such pains. If you are a woman and have any of these pains, you want to have your gallbladder evaluated and should also consider some dietary restrictions to prevent gallbladder attacks.

c. Menstruation

Lower back pain accompanying menstruation is caused by contractions in the uterus. Every month a woman's body builds up a thick uterine lining in preparation for a fertilized egg. If the fertilized egg doesn't arrive, your body will break down and detach the lining by contracting. If the uterus contracts too strongly, it can press on nearby blood vessels, cutting off the supply of oxygen to the nearby muscles, which can lead to pain in the abdomen and the lower back.

Such pain and its underlining cause are often harmless. However, you need to seek care if severe pain persists for more than a few days or your pain level drastically increases.

d. Uterus Problems

Besides possible pain originating from the uterus caused by the menstruation cycle, uterus fibroids can also cause pain in the uterus and manifest in the back. Fibroids are non-cancerous growths in the uterus.

There are three main kinds of fibroids in the uterus:

1. Submucosal fibroids are fibroids that grow into the inner cavity of the uterus and are more likely to cause prolonged, heavy menstrual bleeding.

2. Subserosal fibroids are fibroids that project to the outside of the uterus and can sometimes press on the bladder, causing urinary symptoms. If fibroids bulge from the back of the uterus, they can occasionally press either on the rectum, causing a pressure sensation, or on the spinal nerves, causing a backache.

3. Intramural fibroids are fibroids that grow within the muscular uterine wall. If large enough, they can distort the shape of the uterus and cause prolonged, heavy periods, as well as pain and pressure.

If your back pain is due to uterus fibroids, you will also experience other symptoms, such as:

- Heavy or painful menstrual bleeding,
- Prolonged menstrual periods — seven days or more,
- Pelvic pressure or pain that doesn't go away,
- Spotting or bleeding between periods,
- Frequent urination,
- Enlarged uterus and abdomen,
- Difficulty emptying your bladder,
- Pain consistently with intercourse,
- Constipation, or
- Leg pains.

Seek care about your uterus for possible issue with fibroids, if you experience one or more of the above described symptoms with your back pain.

e. Ovary Problem

Ovarian cysts and tumors can lead to dull pain in lower back.

However, if your pain is indeed caused by ovarian cysts or tumors, it will also come with other symptoms, such as:

- Pain or bloating in the abdomen,
- Difficulty urinating, or frequently needing to urinate,
- Pain during sexual intercourse,
- Painful menstruation and abnormal bleeding,
- Weight gain,
- Nausea or vomiting, or
- Loss of appetite, feeling full quickly.

Seek medical care, if your pain is in the lower back and is accompanied by one or more of the symptoms above.

f. Cancer

Back pain can be caused by cancers in the colon, rectum, pancreas, or ovary.

Unfortunately, if the back pain is due to cancer, chances are that the cancer has already spread from where it started.

For example, pancreas cancer often does not cause noticeable symptoms until they are large enough to press on nearby nerves to cause pain in the back or belly. Other pancreas cancers may grow around the bile duct and block the flow of bile. This causes, in similar ways as pancreas stone, pain in the back and the skin and the whites of the eyes to yellow. By the time these signs are noticed, the pancreatic cancer has already spread out of its original place and is in an advanced stage.

Beyond pain in the back, cancers often come with more, sometimes easier to notice, symptoms, such as:

- Fever,
- Fatigue,
- Loss of weight,
- Change of skin color and tone
- A lasting headache,
- Changes in bowel and bladder movements,
- Unusual bleeding or discharge,
- A thickening or a lump in the breast or other parts of the body,
- A nagging cough, or
- Difficulty swallowing.

If you have pain in the back, and experience any of the above symptoms, you need to see a doctor quickly.

The above are some example conditions that reside inside the body, but may cause pain in the back. There are a large number of other conditions inside the body that can cause back pain. The discussion in the above section is to show you that the cause of your back pain maybe outside your back and inside your body. Look into your body if your back pain doesn't go away.

5. Causes of Back Pain In Your Head

Pain doesn't always indicate injury. Many pains are the results of emotional stress.

In many cases, back pain is also a result of mental or emotional stress. Some studies show that such stresses, such as those from a job or a dysfunctional family relationship, may be closely correlated with back pain.

A 2005 study conducted with 860 French-speaking Quebec City workers, with nonspecific back pain in a primary care setting, found that psychological distress analysis of their back pain was 82 percent correct, over the two-year assessment.

This result mirrors those of earlier studies with English speaking workers in the States. A 1995 study found "the level of persisting disability (chronic back pain) to depend principally on measures in the psychosocial domain," and that "early identification of psychosocial problems is important in understanding, and hopefully preventing, the progression to chronicity in lower back trouble."

According to a study published in *Spine* in 2008, authors Tim John Sloan, Rajiva Gupta, Weiya Zhang, and David Andrew Walsh found that organic pain beliefs (e.g., that pain necessarily indicates damage) are associated with an increased catastrophizing thinking (thinking that the pain is never going to get better) in patients with chronic lower back pain (LBP), and that addressing these beliefs may help patients better manage their pain and disability.

Many medical professionals, including conventional medical doctors and chiropractic doctors, have identified emotional stress as a key cause for back pain many decades ago. Dr. John Sarno, MD, a Professor of Clinical Rehabilitation Medicine at New York University's School of Medicine, detailed his findings and concept on back pain caused by emotional stress in his book *Mind Over Back Pain* first published in 1984. He coined the term "Tension Myositis Syndrome" (TMS) describing back pain caused by "physiologic alternation in certain muscles, nerves, tendons, and ligaments" due to emotional stress.

Dr. Sarno found the only muscles susceptible to TMS are postural muscles, including muscles in the back of the neck, of the whole back, and of the buttocks. Among all postural muscles, the postural muscles in the lower back to the buttock area are the most susceptible and most frequent targets of TMS. The second most susceptible group of postural muscles are those behind the neck.

Like muscle spasms triggered by leaked content of torn cells, it may be a self-protective mechanism designed by nature for certain muscles, nerves, tendons, and ligaments to sense pain when the subconscious mind believes that certain parts of the back are injured or needs to be protected from further injury.

For example, the thought that an anticipated vacation may

exaggerate an existing back injury may be sufficient to trigger or cause a sensation of pain in that part of the back. TMS may also happen when a person has a strong resentment towards some involuntary duties forced on her or him. It is the body's self-protective mechanism to shut down to prevent it from performing the task her body subconsciously believes she shouldn't do.

The body creates such a protective pain in the associated part of the back by decreasing blood and thus oxygen supply to select muscles, nerves, tendons or ligaments – a condition called Ischemia which often leads to pain, numbness, or weakness in the associated tissue.

In a sense, our back may be a more truthful face to our underlying emotions that we may not be consciously aware of. Our subconscious fear and resentment are manifested as pain, while confidence and bravery often lead to relief and freedom for the back.

This is another indication that you are your spine. Your most critical, self-protective mechanism is built in your back, instead of your arms or your legs.

This is another reason not to be too quick to reach out to pain killers or Nonsteroidal Anti-Inflammatory Drugs (NSAIDs) that are too often prescribed to you when back pain occurs. Our back and its pain are truly a mirror reflecting the underlying issues important to us. It's better to carefully take the warning of the mirror, and find the cause of the problem to protect your body from great harm.

Comparing your back pain to a house fire, by simply smashing the house's fire alarm will not stop the burning of the house. Unfortunately, prescribing or taking pain killers, NSAIDs, topical creams, cold packs, hot blankets, TENS (Transcutaneous Electrical Nerve Stimulation) or massage treatment to cover up the pain, instead of diagnosing and treating the cause of the pain, is precisely the equivalent of "smashing the alarm when house is burning", and has become a dangerously prevalent practice in dealing with back pain.

Respect your back. Respect your back pain. And respect the alarm function of your back pain. Find out what it is trying to tell you and deal with the cause. You will thank yourself down the road.

5

36 Common Misconceptions About Back Pain You Must Break

A large number of back pain related misconceptions that are detrimental to back pain sufferers in their recovery and prevention exist. You'll be able to recognize these easily as we go through them, from your understanding of this book so far.

Go through the following list, to see whether you or those you love have any of these misconceptions. If so, explain to yourself why they are misconceptions, and get rid of them.

Put them behind you. Imagine you are driving a convertible on a beautiful country road. Put all your past misconceptions in a bag and throw it into the air. Watch, in your rear-view mirror, the bag dropping on the road behind you, becoming smaller and smaller, disappearing and vanishing completely, behind you. ... By doing so, you will gain a new and stronger mind and confidence to deal with your back problems in the future.

The top 35 misconceptions that back pain sufferers have:

1. Look ma, my back pain is gone. I am all cured now!

2. Bed rest is good for recovery from back pain.

3. Resting in a chair helps recover from back pain.

4. Movement can worsen back pain.

5. Severe back pain can paralyze my spine.

6. I have back pain, it must mean that there is something seriously wrong with me.

7. Taking painkillers is the right thing to do.

8. Visiting my family doctor should be the first thing to do when back pain hits.

9. Conventional medicine is more effective to back pain than non-conventional medicine.

10. As cold or heat packs, massage, and topical creams relieve back pain, they must cure the problem.

11. If I don't lift heavy objects, back pain won't happen to me.

12. I have a comfortable chair at work; so back pain won't affect me.

13. I know how to walk in high heels, so back pain won't strike me.

14. I am muscular and strong; so back pain won't happen to me.

15. I exercise regularly; so back pain won't hit me.

16. I am a tough guy, back pain is nothing to worry about. I don't need to do anything to prevent it.

17. Back pain only happens to older people.

18. Back pain is inherited, no one in my family has it, therefore I won't have it.

19. I am young, spinal degeneration won't happen to me.

20. Intensity of back pain correlates to the level of damage to my back.

21. X-rays, MRIs, or CT scans can tell what causes my back pain.

22. I am struck with back pain, so I'd better change job or stay away from work.

23. Chronic back pain is caused by stress or depression. The pain will stop once the stress or depression is resolved.

24. Back pain often leads to disability.

25. If no cause is found, I must have a psychological issue that causes the back pain.

26. I have to live with my back pain for the rest of my life.

27. Severe back pain indicates that I need surgery.

28. Prolonged, chronic back pain indicates that I need surgery.

29. If none of the things I have tried work, I need surgery.

30. Surgery is the ultimate cure for back pain.

31. Poor posture, body mechanics and spinal alignment do not always cause back pain, therefore I don't need to pay attention to my posture, my body mechanics and my spinal alignment.

32. Big and cushy executive chairs are good for your back.

33. Chiropractic treatment is dangerous.

34. Surgery cures all.

35. Fluffy sleeping pillows are good for you.

36. Soft mattresses are good for your back.

PART TWO
THE SECRET OF YOUR BACK
- WHAT MAKES IT HAPPY

Read this chapter if you are in pain and are looking for the right care or effective solutions to your back problems quickly.

1

3 Reasons Why Your Current First Line of Defense For Back Pain Is Wrong

Most back pain sufferers are faced with a confusing list of options, and are confused as to what may be the right solution to their problem or what discipline of health care professionals they should see. A 2013 Consumer Report survey showed that its 14,000 respondents tried an average of five or six different treatments over the course of only one year.

The internet offers a vast body of unstructured information. Friends and families offer bits and pieces of often isolated stories. Most healthcare professionals would say you have come to the right place for your back problems, whether you've gone to conventional doctors, osteopathic doctors, chiropractic doctors, physiotherapists, massage therapists, acupuncturists, and even nutritionists.

The reality is that back pain has a large number of possible causes. Each discipline of healthcare providers has its own special set of strengths and weaknesses. Each discipline is best to treat a select range of back pain only. No one discipline can treat all back pain or spinal disorders.

Conventional medicine is an effective, and often indispensible, method of care for spinal damage involving vertebral fracture, and back pain involving serious inflammation or issues with inner organs. However, it is not a solution for all back pain.

Conventional medicine tends to lose its shine if a patient's back pain is caused by a twisted joint, a strained muscle, or a pinched nerve.

Chiropractic medicine is often effective in treating back pain caused by a spinal joint lesion, a pinched nerve or a strained muscle. However, it would have no solution if a patient's pain is caused by a sheared spinal disc (spondylolisthesis, often in L5/S1 or L4/L5 joints), mental pressure, emotional stress, or a serious medical condition, such as cancer.

Physiotherapy may be ideal for patients whose back pain is caused by a pulled muscle, however, would be useless if the patient's back pain is caused by misaligned vertebrae.

Massage therapy may be helpful if the back pain is caused by spasms, however, it's little help if the back pain is caused by a pinched nerve.

Emotional or psychological therapy may be helpful if the back pain is caused by emotional stress, however, it would be a waste of time and money for back pain caused by a spinal joint dysfunction or a serious medical condition, such as cancer.

The correct first point of care is critical in the speed, success and satisfaction of your back and back pain recovery.

Unfortunately, the steps most people take, when hit by back pain, are not right to their particular conditions because of the following reasons.

1. Primary Care Doctors Ranked the Last

While most people go to see a conventional medical doctor or a specialist first when afflicted by back pain, conventional medicine may not be the right choice for you. In fact, it is not the right choice for most back pain cases.

In a 2013 report "Relief for Your Aching Back - What Worked for Our Readers," the Consumer Reports Health Ratings Center surveyed more than 14,000 subscribers who experienced lower-back pain in the past year but never had back surgery. The survey found that: "When back pain goes on and on, many people go to see a primary-care doctor. While this visit may help rule out any serious underlying disease, a surprising number of the lower-back-pain sufferers we surveyed said they were disappointed with what the doctor could do to help."

The report further found that these back pain sufferers were most satisfied with treatments by Chiropractic doctors, while least satisfied with treatments by conventional medical doctors. Below is the satisfaction rating by caregiver from the report.

The percentage of people highly (completely or very) satisfied with their back-pain treatments and advice varied by practitioner visited.

Professionals provided care	*Percent of patients highly satisfied with care*
Chiropractor	59%
Physical therapist	55%
Acupuncturist	53%
Physician, specialist	44%
Physician, primary-care doctor	34%

Source: Consumer Reports Health Ratings Center

Fig. 2.1

According to the American College of Physicians, most general practitioners would recommend one of the few things below:

- Prescribe pain killers or NAIDS (anti-inflammatory drugs),
- Advise rest well and do nothing,
- Prescribe X ray or MRI scans, and/or
- Refer to physiotherapy treatments.

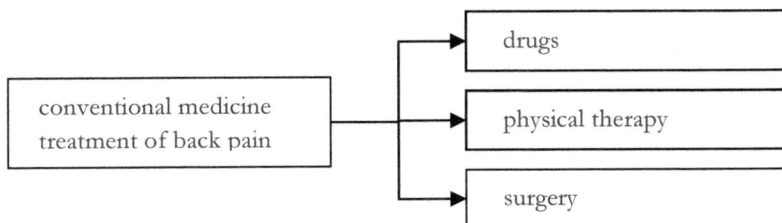

Source: compiled by Patrick Lee

Fig. 2.2

Unfortunately, pain killers mostly serve as a patch only. If you want to mask your pain and consider your problem gone, you don't even need to trouble a doctor. You can simply go to a drug store and buy a pack of pain killers. If you have to see a doctor for strong pain killers because over-the-counter pain killers won't work for you, it may be a strong indication that you need to be serious to ascertain the real cause for your back pain instead of patching it up.

X-ray and MRI scans are expensive, invasive and often of little use in helping diagnose most back pain. If a back pain is not caused by or associated with a condition that causes visible vertebral change in the spine, such as spinal stenosis (the narrowing of the spinal cavity), spondylolisthesis (the forward displacement of a vertebra), arthritis, herniated disc, traumatized vertebrae, severe spinal degeneration, or cancer, X-ray and MRI scans would reveal nothing.

Most back pains are not caused by nor associated with any visible structural change in the spine, rather they may be caused by or associated with repetitive strains of the muscles, minor nerve interference, poor posture and so on.

2. Mismatch of Care for Pain

From the above statistics, where conventional medicine ranked the lowest in patient satisfaction and the description of the treatment approach of conventional medicine, you might begin to think of conventional medicine as being ineffective. Such thinking would be unfortunate.

Conventional medicine not only helps you rule out serious causes, such as inflammation or cancer, but also helps you treat conditions that no other form of medicine or care could be successful at.

One of the main causes for this situation is the fact that, when suffering from back pain, most people first go to a conventional medical doctor, while only a small minority of all back pain cases are suitable to be treated by conventional medicine. Asking an electrician to build a wooden frame, instead of getting a carpenter to do it, will end in disappointment.

Finding the right person to care for you first will dramatically increase your success of recovery and your satisfaction of the care you receive across all above ranges of care. As a patient, you need to take on the responsibility for your own back health, instead of throwing yourself to the care provider that may not be most suitable in your situation. This will reduce your chance of becoming disappointed when the care you received didn't work out as well as expected.

A mismatch of professional care for back pain also results in a misconception about the effectiveness of the available care options.

An unfortunate fact is that 90 percent of back pain sufferers resort to conventional medicine as their first line of defense, while the majority of conventional medicine practitioners are highly limited in their expertise for treating most back pain. Using family doctors as the first line of defense for back pain often leads to unnecessary suffering, frustration, and is a waste of money, time, and opportunity. Is it really the family physicians' fault when patients are disappointed in their treatment for back pain? Isn't it part of patients' responsibility to reach out to the right care at the first place?

In a paper published by the World Health Organization (WHO) in 2003 "Improved Education in Musculoskeletal Conditions Is Necessary for All Doctors," authors Kristina Åkesson, Assistant Professor, University of Lund; and Department of Orthopaedics, Malmö University Hospital, Sweden and her co-authors stated: "Many GPs and family doctors do not have adequate training and consequently lack the competency, skills, and confidence to manage musculoskeletal disorders in their daily practice: they may not recognize conditions or be aware of what can be achieved by appropriate care"

In a 2000 paper "Confidence of Graduating Family Practice Residents in Their Management of Musculoskeletal Conditions," authors JM Matheny, Department of Orthopedic Surgery, Saint Lukes Medical Center, Cleveland, Ohio, USA. and his co-authors pointed out that, in the States, family practice graduates reported a lower level of confidence in their physical examination, radiographic evaluation, diagnosis, and treatment of musculoskeletal patients compared with their confidence levels in dealing with other patients.

3. Ignorance Contributes to the Occurrence, Worsening, Repetition, and Chronicity of Back Pain

The above survey also found that 35 percent of back pain sufferers never consulted a professional. Many of them said it was because they did not think professional care could help. The chances are that your back pain will get better if you find the right care. The key is to find the right care, at least the right starting point, quickly, before suffering too long unnecessarily.

2

6 Reasons Why You Must Be Your Own First Line Of Defense

In today's world, the first line of defense should be you – the back pain sufferer or the individual who wants to prevent back pain. Why? Several reasons:

1. **Conventional Medicine Is Just Too Conventional**
   Conventional medicine does little, except in cases where back pain is caused by other diseases, such as an illness with internal organs, cancer, or vertebral damage, while most back pains are caused by minor mechanical issues.

2. **Everyone's an Expert (While They Aren't)**
   The majority of health care providers you see will tell you that they can treat your problem, while only one or two disciplines of healthcare are truly beneficial to you in your particular case. Most doctors and therapists have good intentions, they want to help you. They are speaking from a sense self-confidence, or professional pride that may or may not be justified, and they may

lack the knowledge needed to really help your specific condition. Then there may be some that are interested in purely financial gain earned from your business.

3. **Professional Training Limitations**
Due to limitations in professional knowledge or experience, your doctor may recommend you for spinal surgery for a condition which actually does not need such an invasive treatment. According to Dr. Nancy Epstein, a highly regarded spinal neurosurgeon: "over the course of the years, I looked at all of the patients with neck and back complaints coming in who were told they needed surgery. And out of those, at least a third of those (who had been) scheduled for operations, I didn't think they needed it (the surgery)." Family doctors often lack knowledge and expertise for back pain or spinal issues. You should see an expert that specializes in spinal health and back pain treatment.

4. **Misdiagnosis**
According to Jerome Groopman, a professor of medicine at Harvard University and the author of the best-selling *How Doctors Think*: "18-seconds is the average time it takes for a doctor to interrupt you as you're describing your symptoms. By that point, your doctor has in mind what the answer is, and he or she is probably right about 80 percent of the time." In other words, one in every five cases is misdiagnosed, or you have a 20 percent chance of being misdiagnosed.

5. **Professional Bias**
Doctors and therapists are humans too. Like all professions, they also have a professional bias. Because they know their own discipline the most, they may occasionally overestimate the effectiveness of their own approach and underestimate those of the alternative healthcare professions. For example, a surgeon may believe an operation the best solution for you.

"Surgeons are doers," says Dr. Nancy Epstein, a spinal neurosurgeon. "If there is a problem, we want to solve the problem. But one of the most difficult things to do is to recognize when we are not the right one to solve the problem.

We have to stand back and not operate. And then refer these patients to another one of our colleagues who are going to do better in terms of treating them non-surgically"

"Far too many patients are having operations that they don't need" she continued. "And these are associated with severe complications including long-term disability or even death."

This phenomenon is also applicable to other health care professionals, such as chiropractors, physiotherapists, and massage therapists. To someone with a hammer, (especially those slightly lacking in knowledge and expertise), everything looks like a nail. You don't want to become the wrong nail to a hammer.

6. **Professional Competence**
   Like high school graduates, some doctors and therapists receive their healthcare license with full marks in their licensing exams and continuing educations, while some barely pass the required exams or made the minimum hours of continuing education. There is a significant gap in the professional capacity among various practitioners.

   You must be your own first line of defense. You must learn whom to seek for healthcare when afflicted by back pain. Otherwise you may endure unnecessary suffering, waste hard earned money, and lose the best window of opportunity for your recovery.

   You may say: "I am too busy and don't have time to learn about the spine and back pain." It is at your peril. If you don't have time for your back, your back will not have time for you when you need it, and often at the most critical moment.

   You may say: "I am not a doctor and don't want to become a doctor." Well, you don't need to become a doctor. You only need to know so much to intelligently chose your healthcare provider and have an informed discussion with her/him for the best possible outcome.

   For those who want to take an active role in their own back health, the following is a road map designed to help you quickly find the most effective care, to reduce suffering, and save time and money.

However, you must be warned, that this road map is not designed for self-diagnosis or self-treatment of your back pain. It is purely designed to help you to quickly identify the most suitable starting point of care for your back when hit by pain.

3

10 Cornerstones of Your Back Pain Strategy

There is a wide range of relief and treatment options available to most back pain sufferers. However, before we dive into the specifics of the wide range of options, you may want to take the following general guidelines into consideration, and carefully follow them.

Here are 10 cornerstones you must incorporate into your back pain strategy:

1. Stay Away from Drugs as Much as You Can

Drugs and other superficial pain killing solutions, ad discussed earlier, may fool you into thinking the underline issues of your back pain is cured because you are not feeling your pain, while they may even be intensifying or getting worse. As a result, they may mislead you, causing you to ignore the underlying cause of the pain, or even to start engaging in physical activities that actually worsen your condition. This could slow your recovery, or even make your condition become chronic.

A fresh coat of paint does not stop a rotten wood from continued rotting underneath. Patching up the pain only hides the real cause of your pain, which you can only understand from a critical examination.

2. Identify and Treat the Cause of Your Back Pain

Some of the causes to back pain are not easy to identify. However, as discussed before, for sustainable relief or prevention of repetition, you must work with your doctor to identify the true cause and treat it accordingly. You must be patient with your doctor, and don't press for immediate pain relief. Otherwise, you may end up silencing your fire alarm while letting your house continue to burn, unknowingly, unnecessarily, and undesirably.

Please see: "A Quick Roadmap For First Care," later in this chapter to help you identify which type of doctors or therapists may be in the best position to help you identify the true cause of your particular pain and condition quickly.

3. Help Your Doctor Identify the True Cause for You

Doctors are busy people. To make sure that you get the right diagnosis, you must become their partner, working with them, instead of simply throwing yourself at your doctor and saying: "diagnose me." You must first find the right doctor to work with who is in the best position to provide you with the right diagnosis. You then must prepare for your visit to your doctor's office to be able to provide the right information in a concise way. You must also ask the right questions to help your doctor avoid misdiagnosis.

For help in quickly and effectively partnering with your doctors for a successful management of your back pain, please refer to the:

- "4 Secrets Helping You Avoid Wrong Doctors" section of this book,
- "8 Things You Could Do To Help Your Doctor Minimize The Risk of Misdiagnosis" section of this book,
- and the lists of questions you should ask your doctor, at the end of this chapter.

4. Don't Rush to MRI or X-ray Scans

Too much Magnetic Resonance Imaging (MRI) magnetism and X-ray radiation is not good for your health. And the causes of most back pain can't be detected via such procedure.

The American College of Physicians (ACP) has officially recommended that doctors stop and think before ordering diagnostic imaging, such as lumbar radiography, Computed Tomography (CT scans), and MRI scans, for patients with lower back pain.

Diagnostic imaging often reveals no abnormal condition among back pain sufferers, even those who may suffer from severe lower back pain.

In front of trained eyes, diagnostic imaging can reveal a wide range of changes in the skeletal structure of the spine, such as a bone fracture, a bone dislocation, spinal degeneration, spinal stenosis, spondylolisthesis, or a herniated disc. However, diagnostic imaging often is not capable of revealing any soft tissue injury or mild to medium spinal joint lesions, which are often the main cause of back pain.

Research shows that unnecessary diagnostic imaging drives up health care costs and has little value for most patients. The tests might cause harm through unnecessary radiation exposure and lead to more tests or invasive procedures that fail to ease symptoms.

"They do not improve patient outcomes and may increase the risk of cancer, especially in women," said Amir Qaseem, MD, PhD, director of clinical policy with the ACP's medical education division.

Authors of ACP's *Annals of Internal Medicine* analyzed six randomized trials that included 1,804 patients who had primarily acute or subacute lower back pain and no evidence of an underlying condition. However, they couldn't find any difference in pain, function, quality of life or overall improvement between patients who underwent imaging tests and those who did not. No difference was reported in patients who received radiography versus advanced imaging tests, such as MRI and CT scans.

5. Keep in Motion By Exercising

Back pain often involves both primary and secondary sources. Often the best treatment can only be provided by you – the patient. Staying active and keeping your body moving is one of the best things you can do to help your body in its recovery from pain, as long as the activities and exercises do not significantly exaggerate your existing back pain. You should stop or reduce your exercise immediately if you feel the extra pain after a night of sleep.

Keeping motion in your body is critical in reducing and

preventing muscle spasms that create pain – the pain from the secondary source, which often can be more severe than the pain from the primary source.

Motion in the back helps prevent deep stabilizing muscles from tensing and will help relieve back pain. Any gentle exercise involving the back are very helpful. Walking is an ideal exercise, because it not only helps pull you out of your bed or chair, but also helps you to maintain a better posture and keep the motion in your back. However, one should avoid any exercise or activity that forces the back in one static position for a prolonged period, such as gardening, crafting, or even web-surfing.

It's a common myth to think movement will further damage your back. Many people have such a fear. There is even a condition called Fear Avoidance Syndrome. The chart below illustrates how this self-re-enforcing pain circle works.

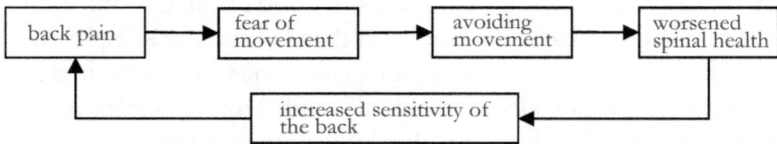

Source: compiled by Patrick Lee

Fig. 2.3

Back pain causes a fear of movement because the sufferer believes that moving makes the pain worse or further damages the back or spine. With this fear, the sufferer begins to reduce, minimize or avoid physical movements. Lack of movement in the back allows further progression of the tension and spasms in the muscles surrounding the injured, inflamed or irritated joints or tissues. Such lack of movement also contributes to:

- Reduced blood circulation to the affected muscles,
- Slowed healing of the muscles, if they were injured,
- Worsened hydration and nutrition supplies to the spinal discs.

These make the spine more susceptible to damage, injury, or pain. As a result, back pain becomes more present, even more intense. Such results further increases the fear of movement, and the vicious circle continues.

6. Limit bed rest and sitting still on couches or chairs.

When afflicted with back pain, the first thing a suffering person would like to do is rest. To lie down on a bed, or to take a seat on a chair, a couch or a recliner. However, sitting on a couch, a chair or a recliner significantly compromises the sufferer's posture and spinal alignment, and reduces blood circulation in the back.

Also physical inactivity often leads to unnecessary contracting or stiffening of the affected back muscles, which tends to worsen the pain at hand. The softer the bed or sitting surface, the more compromised the sufferer's posture is, the more physically inactive the sufferer's body becomes, the worse the back pain tends to become, and the slower the recovery process becomes. To sit on a soft couch is one of the worst things a back pain sufferer could do.

Long distance travel should be avoided. Prolonged sitting in cars or on airplanes is detrimental to the recovery of back pain, because of worsened posture, spinal alignment, and blood circulation.

People with short-term lower back pain who remain physically inactive for prolonged time often feel more pain and have a harder time with daily tasks than those whose backs stay active. Gentle ongoing physical activity to the lumbar back will help you better cope with back pain.

Even a back surgery should not hold you back from movement for too long. After a surgery: "patients should avoid more than three days of bed rest," says orthopedic surgeon Mike Flippin, MD, who specializes in back and spine care at the San Diego Medical Center. "I encourage my patients to get moving as quickly as possible."

7. **Maintain Good Posture**

The majority of back pain is mechanical in nature. With good posture, your spine is properly aligned, your chest is open, and your ligaments and muscles are kept in good tone. With poor posture, your spine is misaligned, your ligaments and muscles are used asymmetrically, excessively and are weakened. Poor posture causes extra stress and tension in the back, and deteriorates the biomechanical condition of the spine.

Hence, activities carried out with a poor posture, such as lifting a heavy weight without maintaining a straight back, or sitting in front of a computer with a slumped back are often the causes for mechanical injuries in the back. Likewise, poor posture also exaggerates back pain and hinders its recovery after its onset.

Sitting is more harmful than most people have realized. Even in a good position, the pressure in the spinal vertebrae would double while sitting compared to standing. According to a study published by K. H. E. Kroemer and E. G. Grandjean in 1997, the spinal disc pressure while sitting is 190 percent of that while standing.

Your neck posture is critical to the health of your neck. The pervasive use of computers, smart phones and video games has made Forward Head Posture a health pandemic more prevalent than ever before. A two to three inches of forward head protrusion, (a condition called Forward Head Posture or FHP), increases the stress and tension in the neck muscles by 200 to 300 percent.

More importantly, is the cumulative effect of such extraordinary stresses in the muscles. As is the case of Repetitive Strains Injuries that can happen to neck, shoulder, arm, wrist, hand and back. Repetitive Strains Injuries is also referred as Cumulative Trauma Disorders, Repetitive Stress Injuries, Repetitive Motion Injuries or Disorders, and Occupational or Sports Overuse Syndromes. In Repetitive Strains Injuries, the micro damages including microscopic tears, deprivation of blood circulation, deprivation of lubricant fluid, abnormal abrasion, inflammation, and nerve irritation, to muscles, tendons, and nerves accumulate over time, and may lead to

- pain, aching or tenderness.
- stiffness.
- throbbing.
- weakness.
- cramp
- tingling or numbness.

As one ages, the speed of muscle regeneration and recovery slows down. Once the speed of muscle recovery is lower than the rate of the cumulative growth rate of the micro damages, the repetitive strain injury occurs. Harmless sitting becomes the silent killer of your back.

Furthermore, good posture increases your vital capacity and overall strength and the speed of your neuromuscular system to regenerate.

8. Stay Away from Braces As Much as Possible

Braces can both immobilize and weaken your muscles. Immobilization may exaggerate your pain. And weakening your muscles may increase the risk of future reoccurrence of your pain. While a brace may be tempting, you should use it as little and as brief as possible. It may be the wrong reason for using a brace temporarily while doing something that may be too strenuous during your recovery, because you should avoid performing such activities in the first place.

Always think in the long-term interest of your body. The sky will not fall if some task is left undone or is left to others to do. If you absolutely have to perform the task and must use the brace, use it for no more than 20-minutes, which also means that you should really take a break no more than 20-minutes into the strenuous task.

Remember, if the rate of ongoing damage is higher than the recovery rate of your muscles you are making your condition worse.

Also remember:

- Cheaper treatments are often better.
- Take it easy for a day or two.
- Get a second doctor's opinion, especially from a professional of a different discipline.

9. Get Help from Your Friends

Your friends and loved ones who have had similar issues before can be a great source of help to you. Ask them for their experience, advice, and referrals.

If no one you know have had similar issues before, ask them about their family and friends. You can also contact special interest groups locally or online. The members of such groups will often readily discuss with you your concerns and share with you their experiences, and offer their recommendations. Their referrals can also be very helpful.

10. Go with the Least Invasive Care First

Unless you know that you have a freshly fractured vertebra, or a cancer that is the cause of your pain, stay away from an invasive treatment. The more invasive the potential solution is, the more time you need to think it over and the more people you need to consult before you commit to it.

Do not be pressured into surgery. In the absence of a recent severe trauma, you want to opt to wait for at least several months before making a commitment for surgery if your pain is not life threatening, especially when it is chronic in nature. This is particularly important to younger people because they lack life experience and tend to be easier pressured to commit to invasive solutions.

4

9 Proven Relief Options You Must Consider

There are a wide range of treatments and preventative solutions. Each one has its advantages and disadvantages. It is critical to have a degree of knowledge about how to select the right solution for yourself according to your condition and objective.

"Ah, …" You may say, "I will leave it to my healthcare provider." Unfortunately, back pain is a complex issue for which no single healthcare discipline has all the answers.

As medical science advances, today we have the knowledge about back pain, its treatment, and its prevention that reaches the range and depth that has never been possible or imaginable before.

As a result, back pain treatment and prevention has been divided into a wide range of detailed fine disciplines, branches, principles or schools. Most health care providers tend to specialize in one particular discipline, branch, principle or school. For example, in the USA, osteopathic doctors tend to prescribe surgeries as a means of treatment.

On the other hand, back pain sufferers tend to have a

conventional primary care giver who tends to treat or refer her or his patient to the discipline of care she or he knows best, such as physiotherapy or orthopedic surgery. As a result, you would, figuratively speaking, become a nail, if you see someone with a hammer, which may lead you down the less optimal path of recovery or prevention.

You should always start with the least invasive treatment. You should always exhaust the less invasive treatment before seeking the next more invasive treatment. Intensity of pain has no direct correlation with the invasiveness of a treatment required. Severe pain doesn't mean that you have to jump to highly invasive treatment.

The length or duration of the pain doesn't have a direct correlation with the invasiveness of the treatment required. There is no rule to say the longer your pain persists, the more invasive an approach or a treatment is required.

In general, manual treatments tend to be less invasive than surgeries. And within surgeries, the invasiveness of different approaches varies greatly. And as technology and medical discoveries progress, more and more less-invasive surgeries are becoming available every year. What you heard as the least invasive and most effective approach a year ago, may no longer be the case by the time you consider your options.

At this point, you may say: "well, I am too busy and don't have time to learn about my back." The reality is that the health of your back and spine is the essential condition for your freedom, productivity, and quality of life. If you don't have time for your back now, your back may not have time for you in the future.

Learn about your back health now! Otherwise, you are damaging your back each time you sit, each time you lift a heavy object, each day you go to work, each time you drive a car, each time you watch a TV program, or even each time you go on a vacation! \

The cumulative effect of these daily damages will cause premature degeneration of your spine, cause preventable back suffering, cause preventable productivity decline, cause a foreseeable handicap in your favourite activities, such as golfing, cycling, walking your dog, doing your craft work, or even enjoying your dinner.

All of these are learned, to various degrees via personal suffering by those who had suffered or are suffering from back pain. Those who have not experienced a significant episode of back pain only need to talk to a friend who has. Chances are you don't want to learn about these consequences via your personal suffering. To learn from someone else's knowledge and experiences, instead of via your own body, is a better approach on this topic.

You need to start now! Otherwise, you may have to learn about them through your own pain and suffering. According to the National Institute of Health, over 80 percent of us will experience a significant episode of acute back pain in our life time, and many of those episodes will repeat within a year or so down the road, as discussed before.

"But, it is too late for me to learn now, because I have had back pain for a while and have been under treatment for some time," you may say. Better late than never! Start learning today!

Where do we begin with our discussion of specific options available to back pain sufferers? To be pragmatic, let's follow the order of the form of care most satisfied by the 14,000 participants of the Consumer Reports survey as presented in the earlier part of this book, as discussed in Part Two, Chapter 1.

As an exception, however, ergonomics is placed as the first thing to explore. Because, if your pain is not caused by problems in your inner organs, pathological nerve compression, or is constantly on your mind, no amount of care will help you if you continue to put your body in a condition that may have caused you the pain or problems in the first place, regardless if you spend your day at work or at home.

1. Ergonomics

Back pain is one of the most common work-related injuries and is often caused by ordinary work activities, such as sitting in an office chair or heavy lifting.

In fact, heavy weight lifting and sitting are the top two causes for back pain in North America. Together they cause the majority of back pain each year. A great portion of back pain is caused by poor posture and incorrectly operating tools or performing various duties at work, home, or school.

Ergonomics studies the relation and interaction between people and their tasks, tools, equipment, machines, and supporting facilities, such as chairs, desks, and floors, in a workplace or in a public or a private living environment. Applying ergonomic principles and practices can help reduce and prevent work-related back pain and back injury.

To help you reduce and prevent back injuries or back pains, some important ergonomic tips are below:

- Use your muscles not your bones!

- Use your muscles dynamically instead of statically! (Otherwise, you wear them out, like running an engine without oil.)

- Keep your chest out, chin in, shoulders open, stomach tight, body straight, whenever you can, standing, walking, lifting, bending and sitting.

- Standing: Keep two feet in parallel, shoulder-wide apart, when ironing, washing dishes, or even standing at work.

- Sitting: Use a lumbar support in your car and/or chair or adjust your car seat to a more upright position. Sitting up straight puts the least amount of stress on the spine. It may take more muscular and mental effort, but it is wise to create this new awareness and habit!

- Sleep by lying on the side: Keep the bottom leg straight, while top leg can be bent or rested on pillow.

- Bending: keep your back straight when putting dishes in the dishwasher, getting laundry out of the washer, or putting items into the trunk of your car.

- Lifting: Keep the object being lifted close to you and get down under it.

Remember that chronic poor posture causes a loss of flexibility in the major muscles in front of the shoulders (i.e., the pectoralis major muscle), decreases the mobility of the cervical spine, and causes loss of strength of the scapular muscles, making it almost impossible to maintain good posture.

2. Chiropractic

Back pain, especially lower back pain, treatment is one of the key specialties of Chiropractic medicine. Chiropractic medicine was founded by Canadian American D.D. Palmer in Davenport, Iowa, USA, in 1895.

D.D. Palmer was a healer practicing mesmerism – part of which was the 19th century equivalent of modern day hypnotherapy. Mesmerism was created by German physician Franz Anton Mesmer, due to his success in a hypnosis practice, the word "mesmerize" has been widely used to this day. Hypnosis uses the power of the brain to affect the nervous system.

As a result, D.D. Palmer was very interested in the function of the brain and the nervous system, and its effect on the body. This eventually lead to his success in helping restore the hearing of Harvey Lillard, an African America Janitor who had been deaf for 17-years after a spine injury. As a result, chiropractic medicine was born, and Harvey Lillard was entered into history as the first chiropractic patient.

As its reputation gradually grew for treating back pain, and a wide range of other hard to handle medical conditions without drugs and surgery, chiropractic medicine has become a licensed medical profession with 100,000 practitioners, formally organized in 90 countries around the world.

According to a large scale survey of 14,000 back pain patients by Consumer Reports, chiropractic care was ranked number one in patient satisfaction for back pain treatment.

Treatment	% of patients found helpful
Chiropractic	58%
Spinal injection	51%
Massage	48%
Physiotherapy	46%
Prescription medication	45%
Over the counter medication	22%

Source: Consumer Report survey 2013
Fig. 2.4

After traditional medicine, most back pain sufferers choose chiropractic treatment in the USA. About 22 million Americans visit chiropractors annually. After trying a range of, often 5 to 6 various back pain relief treatments, most patients would favor hands-on manual treatments with chiropractic care as their top choice. Chiropractic care truly deserves to be a top choice for back pain sufferers.

According to Dr. Melinda Ratini, DO, Lower Bucks Hospital and WebMD, most people seeking back pain relief alternatives choose chiropractic treatment. 22 million Americans visit chiropractors annually. 35% of them are seeking relief from back pain.

"Studies suggest that people who have back pain for at least two weeks and are not getting better are the ones who get the most benefit from chiropractic," said Dr. Ralph E. Gay, MD, physical rehabilitation, Mayo Clinic. "Overall, for the lumbar spine and lower back, it (chiropractic care) is a safe therapy. And it is one with more random trials and more studies behind it than any of the other integrative therapies that we use for back pain."

Chiropractors use manual spinal manipulation with hands or various powered or non-powered instruments. Chiropractic physicians believe that proper alignment of the body's musculoskeletal structure, particularly the spine, will help the body to reduce or eliminate interference to its nervous system, giving the body a chance to better function and better heal itself, often without surgery or medication.

As conventional physicians frequently reach out to prescribing drugs and surgeries, chiropractic physicians often prefer the less invasive approach -- treatment without drugs and surgeries. Each has its advantages and disadvantages. In many instances, patients receive a combination of chiropractic and traditional medical care.

While the professional title for a traditional physician is "Medical Doctor" or "MD," the professional title for a chiropractic physician is "Doctor of Chiropractic" or "DC." A Doctor of Chiropractic also attends specialized post-secondary schooling, whose education typically includes an undergraduate degree plus four years of chiropractic college.

As traditional physicians use many different medicines to treat their patients, chiropractic physicians use a wide range of "techniques" and instruments to treat their patientsThe following are the top fifteen most widely applied Chiropractic techniques, according to Job Analysis of Chiropractic, by the National Board of Chiropractic Examiners in January 2000.

Technique/Procedure	% of DC Use
1. Diversified	95.9%
2. Extremity manipulating/adjusting	95.5%
3. Activator Methods	62.8%
4. Gonstead	58.5%
5. Cox Flexion/Distraction	58.0%
6. Thompson Technique	55.9%
7. Sacro Occipital Technique	41.3%
8. Applied Kinesiology	43.2%
9. NIMMO/Receptor Tonus	40.0%
10. Cranial	37.3%
11. Adjustive Instruments	34.5%
12. Palmer Upper Cervical	28.8%
13. Logan Basic	28.7%
14. Meric	19.9%
15. Pierce-Stillwagon	17.1%

Source: National Board of Chiropractic Examiners

Fig. 2.5

And the following is a list of other popular chiropractic techniques from the total of close to 100 chiropractic techniques developed in the past 120 years, in alphabetical order.

- Activator Technique
- Active Release Technique
- Applied Kinesiology
- Atlas Orthogonal
- B.E.S.T. (Bio Energetic Synchronization Technique)
- Biomechanics
- Carver Technique
- Chiropractic Biophysics
- Contact Reflex Analysis
- Cox Flexion / Distraction

- Craniosacral Therapy
- Diversified
- Gonstead
- Graston Technique
- Impulse Adjusting Technique
- Logan Basic
- Motion Palpation
- Network
- Neuro Muscular Technique
- Pettibon
- Sacral Occipital Technique (SOT)
- Soft Tissue Orthopedics
- Spinal Biomechanics
- Thompson
- Traction
- Upper Cervical Specific
- Versendaal

Each technique has its own specific strengths and benefits, and is specially effective to certain conditions. There is no one technique that could be suitable to all back pain cases. Most doctors could excel in only three to four different techniques. There is no one doctor who is a master of all of these special techniques.

It is important for back pain patients to understand the fact that there is a wide range of chiropractic techniques, research and experiment with various techniques to find the ones most effective and suitable to your specific situation.

Chiropractic doctors also use a range of assistive therapeutic tools, which are often referred to as modalities. Most frequently used may be laser devices, infrared devices, and spinal decompression equipment.

The following is a list of the most common chiropractic instruments:

- Laser,
- Mechanical vibrators, adjustors,
- Tens units,
- Spinal decompression,

- Traction devices,
- Nutrition,
- Infrared, and
- Massage.

Like chiropractic techniques, no one modality could be effective and suitable to all back pain cases. It is also a matter of trying and experimenting with different modalities to find the most effective one for you.

A chiropractic treatment plan may involve one or more manual adjustments, in which the doctor manipulates the joints or soft tissues using varied, yet controlled force to improve range and quality of motion, and reduce or eliminate nerve interference. Many chiropractors also incorporate laser, infrared, spinal decompression, nutritional counseling, acupuncture, massage, and rehab exercises into the treatment plan. The goals of chiropractic care include the restoration and revitalization of function, improved overall health and wellbeing, and prevention of injury, in addition to back pain relief. Chiropractic aims to resolve the root cause of the suboptimal health, functional disorder or bodily pain.

While the general public may have some degree of misunderstanding about it, chiropractic treatment is one of the most effective, least invasive, and safest forms of treatment or care of spinal health or back pain.

Based on the four separate studies of D. J. Henderson, P. Jaskoviak, A. G. Terrett, and B. Lauretti, the death rate related to chiropractic neck manipulation is less than one in a million. While there are no deaths reported with other chiropractic manipulations, such as lower back or extremity manipulations.

On the other hand, a Finnish study using data from the Finnish PERFECT-back database (data collected from a hospital discharge register) found that a total of 408 (0.67%) patients died during the first year after surgery, from a total of 61,166 patients who had undergone surgery for a degenerative spine condition between 1997 and 2009.

These patients either had a herniated lumbar disc, spinal stenosis, degenerative disc disease, spondylolysis, or spondylolisthesis. The lead author of the study, Jyrki Salmenkivi (Helsinki University Central Hospital, Espoo, Finland), commented at Euro Spine 2013: "Death because of medical error was utterly rare. Only one person died directly because of surgery." As a result, the study indicates that the death rate directly related to surgery was one out of 61,166. Certainly one may argue that the patients who underwent surgery have conditions more severe than those that only received chiropractic care. Unfortunately, there exists no data that would support a direct apple to apple comparison. However, it is reasonable to assume that chiropractic care is no more risky than surgery.

And it is in your best interest to look into chiropractic care as a potential option for treating your back pain or spinal disorder. This may not only save you much pain and money, but also save the health care system much capacity and cost.

Since chiropractic does not use drugs or apply surgeries, it wouldn't be a good choice for any condition that involves severe inflammation or destruction of bodily parts, such as a broken bone or a torn ligament.

3. Physiotherapy

Physiotherapy or physical therapy is the remediation of impairments and disabilities and the restoration or improvement of mobility, range of motion, degree of flexibility, level of function, and level of independence.

Physiotherapy is often the first care referred to by family physicians for patients with lower back pain, before considering other more aggressive treatments, including back surgery. This initial treatment often lasts four-weeks and focuses on decreasing back pain, increasing range of motion, and preventing future back problems. But it is not necessarily focused on treating the cause of the back pain.

Physical therapies can be divided into two main categories:

1. **Passive Physical Therapy**: This includes therapies and exercises done to the patient who receive these treatments passively without active involvement, such as heat application, ice packs, electrical stimulation and motion exercises.

2. Active Physical Therapy: This focuses on the patient

performing specific exercises and stretching. Active exercises are most commonly used for lower back pain treatment in Active Physical Therapy programs.

Physiotherapists help patients better understand, apply and perform stretching and strengthening to help reduce pain and the inflammatory cycle and accelerate tissue healing. Like chiropractors and ergonomists, they educate the patient on proper posture and ergonomic principles to preserve the spine.

By introducing specific exercises with varied intensity, repetition and frequency, physiotherapists help patients reduce pain and stiffness to specific regions, strengthen relevant muscles, and shorten the time to return to normal activities.

Physiotherapy covers a vast range of health conditions, of which back pain is only a small branch. As a result, most physiotherapists have limited expertise in treating back pain. They often apply hot and cold therapy and some physical exercises. Hot and cold therapy may be helpful to some acute back pain caused by muscular injury, but is, like a pain killer, mostly a patch approach instead of a therapeutic approach. Physical exercises may be helpful in the rehab phase after the cause of the back pain has been resolved. It does little to resolve any cause of back pain, unless the issue is muscular in nature.

4. Acupuncture and Acupressure

Acupuncture and acupressure have been practiced to relieve pain and treat various diseases in China for over 2,000 years, and have become a popular common practice in Western countries. The earliest written record of acupuncture is found in the Huangdi Neijing (The Yellow Emperor's Inner Canon), dated approximately 200 BC.

Acupuncture is so effective in pain relief that it is sometimes used as the only pain relief solution during surgical operations. Best of all, it is virtually free of side effects, unlike any chemical based anesthesia or pain management solutions.

It is not too surprising that it is highly beneficial to back pain sufferers. A study published in the Archives of Internal Medicine in 2009 found that acupuncture helped relieve chronic back pain better than standard care, such as hot and cold packs, medications, or physical therapy.

Interestingly, a simulating acupuncture technique using toothpicks to poke the skin instead of puncture the skin and flesh worked better than the usual care given for the problem, shown by the study.

"Acupuncture-like treatments had a positive effect overall on people's chronic back pain," said study author Dan Cherkin, PhD, at Group Health Center for Health Studies in Seattle. "It didn't matter if you inserted the needle or superficially poked [the skin]."

The study randomly assigned 638 men and women, aged 18 through 70-years-old, with chronic lower back pain who had never before had acupuncture into four groups:

1. Individualized Acupuncture Group, with each patient receiving individually prescribed acupuncture treatments,

2. Standardized Acupuncture Group, with each patient receiving a standard acupuncture treatment designed for chronic lower back pain,

3. Simulated Acupuncture Group, with each patient receiving a treatment that used a toothpick to mimic the needle but without penetrating the skin

4. Usual Care Group, with each patient continuing whatever they were doing previously, such as applying hot and cold packs, taking pain medicine or undergoing physical therapy.

Acupuncture treatments were given two times a week for three weeks, then once a week for four weeks. The researchers measured "pain-bothersomeness" on a zero to ten-point scale and back pain related dysfunction on a 0 to 23-point scale at 8, 26 and 52 weeks after the treatments. The dysfunction measure reflects a patient's ability to engage in activities of daily living, such as going to social functions or performing household tasks.

Eight weeks after the treatments, those who received the acupuncture treatments reported doubled dysfunction improvement over those getting their usual care -- a 4.4 points improvement on the dysfunction scale compared with 2.1 points. The acupuncture treated patients were also more likely to obtain meaningful improvement on the dysfunction scale -- 60 percent of acupuncture treated compared with just 39 percent of the usual care group patients.

Those who received the acupuncture treatments also reported more than double the improvement on the pain relief scale over those getting their usual care -- 1.6 to 1.9 points compared with only

0.7 points.

Even after a year, those in the acupuncture groups were still more likely than the usual-care group to continue their improvement in dysfunction -- 59 to 65 percent of the acupuncture-treated patients compared with 50 percent of the usual care patients.

However, there were no marked differences in incremental benefits between the individualized, the standard, and the simulating acupuncture group. "The individualized acupuncture did not provide any benefit over the standardized acupuncture," Cherkin tells WebMD. "The simulated acupuncture, which did stimulate the standardized points, also had the same effect. All three did better than the usual care group."

In addition, several well-designed European trials have suggested that real acupuncture and simulated acupuncture (e.g., shallow needling of points which is often considered ineffective) are equally effective, and both superior to best practice medical care.

What can be said for sure is that acupuncture works, and it works better than conventional care methods, whether the acupuncture uses individualized, standard or simulating techniques.

The fact that even simulated acupuncture is capable of providing great results shows that acupuncture doesn't always have to involve needles, which is why the ancient acupressure and the modern laser acupuncture have also proven to be effective in treating illness and relieve pain.

All of these techniques are about stimulating the nerves at certain points on or in our body. They may be working with the same sensory receptors, such as the mechanical nociceptor that respond to excess pressure or the mechanical deformation in or on our body. Such receptors may have functions to interfere, interact, or influence the function or physiology of other systems of our body.

The fact that, in this particular study, the various techniques did not show a difference in effectiveness should be taken with a grain of salt. Generally speaking, acupuncture is an art and a science that the science itself has yet to explain fully. Due to the significant physical, physiological, and neurological differences between patients, not only different acupuncture points will result in a different effectiveness, even the depth of penetration, the angle of penetration, and the rotation or temperature of the needle will also result in a different effectiveness, which is why true acupuncture masters have that golden touch that can could resolve a difficult condition within a short period, while others have to take more time and may not be able to deliver a striking result.

The good news is that you don't need a prescription or referral to see a chiropractor, a physiotherapist, or a massage therapist, let alone other manual or naturalistic healing solutions, such as yoga, tai chi, Pilates professionals and so on.

5. Osteopath

Osteopathy was founded by Andrew Taylor Still, MD in the United States in 1874. "Osteo" means "bone" in Latin. Osteopath is so named as Dr. Still believed that: "the bone, osteon, was the starting point from which [he] was to ascertain the cause of pathological conditions."

Dr. Still founded the American School of Osteopathy (now A.T. Still University of the Health Sciences) and insisted on a distinguished professional title "DO" – for "Doctors of Osteopathy Medicine" from "MD," due to his dissatisfaction with the limitations of conventional traditional medicine at the time.

Many osteopaths are also traditional medicine doctors, and carry both DO and MD as their professional titles. Some are also trained in chiropractic and carry more titles such DO, DC, and MD.

Osteopathy emphasizes the interrelationship between musculoskeletal structure and function of the body, as well as the body's ability to heal itself. Dr. Still believed disease was a result of the failure of the body's normal defense systems or homeostatic nature. He believed that an illness is less because of the germ invading the body, but more because of the breakdown of the body's innate capacity to defend and heal.

Dr. Still said: "Nature furnishes its own serums if we know how to deliver them." He believed that the role of the physicians was not simply to kill the invading germs, but rather to support the body's own natural capability to defend and regain the body's own normal health. He concluded that the musculoskeletal system has an integral and interactive function with all other organ systems.

Traditional osteopathy has four official core principles:

1. The person is a unit, and the person represents a combination of body, mind, and spirit.

2. The body is capable of self-regulation, self-healing, and health maintenance.
3. Structure and function are reciprocally interrelated.
4. Rational treatment is based on an understanding of body unity, self-regulation, and the interrelationship of structure and function.

Traditional osteopathy also has four basic theoretical models:

1. **The Postural Structural Model** -- This model focuses on balance and symmetry of the musculoskeletal system to allow the system to restabilize into its healthiest and most functional pattern. For example, a patient with lower back pain is examined for such factors as: leg length discrepancy; flat or fallen arches; injured or dysfunctional knees, ankles, or hips; disruptions in the normal gait or walking patterns; and overuse or underuse of various muscle and joint patterns.

2. **The Neurological Model** -- This model explores how organ dysfunction can affect the musculoskeletal system and also how the musculoskeletal system interacts with the various organ systems. These interactive processes are referred to as viscerosomatic (the inner organs affecting the musculoskeletal system) and somatovisceral (the musculoskeletal system affecting the inner organs) reflexes.
    a. An example of a viscerosomatic reflex is in a patient suffering shoulder pain caused by an acute gallbladder attack. In such a case, the treatment should be directed towards the gallbladder instead of towards the shoulder.
    b. An example of the somatovisceral reflex is in a patient suffering from constipation caused by acute lower back spasms. In such a case, the muscles of the lower intestine may also go into spasms and create constipation. The treatment needs to be focused on the acute lower back spasm instead of the constipation.

3. **The Respiratory-Circulatory Model** – This model views

musculoskeletal systems as a pump for low-pressure circulation (such as the venous and lymphatic systems). The diaphragm is the main pump in this system. If the diaphragm is not working properly, the body's ability to bring fluids out of the lower extremities will be reduced, and an accumulation of fluid in the lower extremities may develop, and lead to swelling in the legs, and in turn, a compromised immune system. In such case, treatments need to be directed towards the diaphragm, instead of the swelling or the compromised immune system alone.

4. **The Psychobehavioral Model** -- This model examines how psychological issues can affect the musculoskeletal system and also how musculoskeletal dysfunction can create psychological disturbances. Injury to the musculoskeletal system can cause anxiety, even depression in severe cases. Like a physical smile can cheer up a person in her mind, a person who tends to slouch with her shoulders rolled forward and chest closed would also tend to have a flatter emotional tone and less positive outlook, compared to people who stand and sit upright, with shoulders and chest open naturally. Studies have shown that relational turmoil and emotional stress often lead to back pain.

Osteopathic doctors also use a wide range of techniques to treat patients. The following are some of the most common ones:

a. **Soft Tissue Manipulation**

Practitioners apply soft tissue manipulation to evaluate the condition of tissues and to help the body's fluids (such as blood and lymphatic fluid) flow smoothly. Keeping fluids flowing smoothly reduces harmful fluid retention and makes the body's immune system more effective.

b. **Osteopathic Articular Technique**

Practitioners use this technique to reduce muscle spasms and ease neurological irritations around a joint to make joints more mobile and to reduce pain and discomfort around the joint.

c. **Cranial Osteopathy**

This is the most gentle osteopathic technique, and it requires the most experience to perform effectively. Practitioners use this gentle technique to assess, treat, and restore the biorhythm in the patient's head, spinal cord, sacrum, and the rest of the patient's body. The technique is performed by manipulating the patient's skull based on the mobility and sensory capacity of the skull bones and its contents.

d. **Visceral Manipulation**

Osteopathic Manual Practitioners use visceral manipulation to treat organs and viscera of the body, including lungs, heart, liver, spleen, kidneys, stomach, pancreas, intestines, bladder, and uterus.

Osteopaths do not get hold of these organs and manipulate them. Instead, osteopaths gently manipulate the structures and the fascia (connective tissue) that surrounds the corresponding organs to stimulate and effect their function by improving the mobility and/or the blood flow of the organ.

Back pain may originate from a stressed inner organ. Based on a special neuro-relationship between the inner organs and the corresponding parts of the body called Viscerosomatic Reflex. A stressed organ sends its sensory signal to the spinal cord and to the cells in a sensory nerve (instead of a motor nerve), which creates pain in a body part that appears unrelated to the inner organ.

Sometimes that body part is in the back. As a result, the stress of an inner organ can manifest itself as a pain in the back. For example a stressed digestive system can cause back pain. Viscerosomatic reflex is not a one way street. The inner organs affects each other.

Unfortunately, many modern osteopaths have ditched these principles and picked up scalpels instead. This is why it is important for patients to understand that, while each has special strengths, a DO may not be a DO in its traditional sense, especially in the USA.

In the past 100 years, osteopaths have developed a reputation for treating lower back pain with noninvasive approaches. However, particularly in the USA, osteopaths have also developed a reputation for spinal surgery, because here the osteopath has evolved into two main branches – surgical operation oriented versus manual manipulation oriented.

The traditional osteopaths aim to facilitate the healing process, principally by the practice of manual manipulative therapy, while many of the new schools of the USA trained osteopaths specialize in spine surgeries. Outside of the USA most osteopaths are manual practitioners, while inside the USA most of today's osteopaths are spine surgeons. If you are lucky enough to find them, traditional osteopaths are still happy to treat you with the original principles, models, and techniques.

It is important to realize the differences between the two key streams of osteopathic medicine, as one has little interest in the medical approach of the other. One is mainly noninvasive, while the other is invasive on the highest order in most cases.

6. Conventional Medicine – Primary Care Practice

Treatment approaches of conventional primary care practices mainly focus on:

a. Advising patients that most back pain is uncomplicated and self-limited, go back and take some good rest.
b. Prescribing analgesics or anti-inflammatory drugs.
c. Recommending physiotherapy care, modern General Physicians (GPs) may recommend, chiropractic, acupuncture, and massage treatments.
d. Checking for other diseases, such as arthritis or cancer (as cancers especially breast, lung, and prostate cancers are known to spread to the spine) that may cause back pain.
e. Recommending and performing surgery mostly for a fractured or degenerated spine.

One of the disadvantages of conventional medicine in treating back pain is that conventional doctors tend to consider that it is not possible to take the back pain away, if they can't find:
- Anything wrong with your internal organs,
- They can't find any sign of tumor or cancer, or
- They can't find any sign of hard trauma to your back.

They tend to believe that, after whatever treatment you have received, "half of the time you will still have pain, only at a lower level, and not interfering with your job, sleep, recreation, exercises and daily activities." Their objectives are mainly to help reduce your back pain or give you the tools to cope with your back pain. Under the guidance of such thinking, the outlook of your treatment by conventional medicine is not promising, if you want to get rid of your back pain.

Conventional medicine is the best choice for treating back pain whose cause or causes are a tumor, cancer, or issues with the internal organs, or stress in the mind of the patient. Of course, other disciplines of care may also be effective in dealing with back pain caused by issues of internal organs or stresses in the mind. You want to keep your mind open for broader possibilities.

7. Massage Therapy

Massage is one of the oldest healing arts of humanity. It focuses on:

- The manipulation of superficial and deeper layers of muscle and connective tissue,
- To relax the muscles and soft tissues,
- Stimulate fascia,
- Promote circulation,
- Reduce waste products in the muscles,
- Accelerate the healing process, and
- Reduce stress, and enhance function and well-being.

There is a wide range of different schools and techniques for massage therapy.

A 2011 study by the National Center for Complementary and Alternative Medicine of 400 adults with moderate to severe lower back pain, led by Dr. Daniel C. Cherkin, PhD, Associate Director and Senior Scientific Investigator with the Center for Health Studies at Group Health Cooperative in Seattle, showed that participants who have undergone massage treatments achieved greater average improvements in pain relief and functional capacity compared to those who had undergone the usual care, such as taking pain medications or muscle relaxants, seeing doctors or chiropractors, physical therapy, or simply not doing anything. What's most interesting is that the type of massage they received didn't seem to affect the positive result, whether weekly whole-body massages or weekly massages that focused on specific muscle problems around the lower back and hips.

At the end of the 10-week study, 37 percent of patients in the massage groups said their pain was nearly or completely gone, compared to 4 percent in the usual care group.

"We found the benefits of massage are about as strong as those reported for other effective treatments: medications, acupuncture, exercise, and yoga," Dr. Cherkin said. "And massage is at least as safe as other treatment options. So people who have persistent back pain may want to consider massage as an option."

For a treatment that doesn't involve the application of chemicals and scalpels, 37 percent of efficacy rate is very high, considering that the flu vaccine that we take each year has an efficacy rate of roughly 50 percent.

According to the Personalized Medicine Coalition, the efficacy rate of many critical drugs still has much room to improve (efficacy rate):

Type of drugs	efficacy rate
Cancer drugs:	25%
Alzheimer drugs:	30%
Arthritis drugs:	50%
Diabetes drugs:	57%
Asthma drugs:	60%
Anti-depressant drugs:	62%

Source: compiled by Patrick Lee

Fig. 2.6

8. Psychosomatic Medicine / Behavioral Medicine

We often speak of how mind and body interact with each other. Studies have repeatedly shown back pain is often associated with a person's mental and emotional state. Mind-body approaches can be highly effective in treating back pain.

This is where psychosomatic medicine and its modern sibling, behavioral medicine, come in. They specialize in treating disorders in which mental factors play a significant role in the development, expression, or resolution of a physical illness.

Psychosomatic medicine can be traced back to ancient Persian psychologist-physicians Ahmed ibn Sahl al-Balkhi and Haly Abbas. They developed an understanding on how a patient's physiology and psychology can affect each other. Back pain and high blood pressure are typical examples that can be traced back to one or more psychological and/or sociological stressor or stressors.

Modern brain imaging of pain provides deeper insights into the nature of pain in the 1990s. New research finds that pain stimulation not only manifests itself in areas of the brain responsible for pain stimulation, but also many other brain areas, which has led to the new concept of a "Pain Neuromatrix."

This new concept underscores the notion that pain is due to the activity and interaction of widely distributed brain regions, and also underscores the notion that pain is due to activity and interaction of widely distributed stressors.

The concept helped practitioners and researchers better understand how sensory, cognitive, affective, behavioral, social, and cultural factors and stress-related phenomena can influence pain. It also showed the possibility that pain could be better managed by modifying the activities in various brain regions through novel biomedical or behavioral interventions.

Chronic pain management is a key field of application of psychosomatic and behavioral medicines. The biopsychosocial model of pain and a pain neuromatrix model have proven to be particularly effective in pain management. Based on these models, pains are affected by three categories of factors:

1. Biological
2. Psychological
3. Social

Psychosomatic and behavioral medicines are not only effective for non-malignant (non-disease caused) chronic back pain, but also effective for malignant (disease caused, such as cancer, osteoarthritis, or rheumatoid arthritis) chronic back pain experience and management.

Psychological factors that affect pain include:

- Self-coping strategies for the pain,
- Self-confidence in managing the pain,
- Pain-related anxiety,
- Fear of pain,
- Fear of movement,
- Depression,
- Emotion,

- Sexual and physical abuse,
- Work stress,
- Relationship stress,
- Life stress,
- Pain belief,
- Pain acceptance,
- Pain catastrophizing
- Social support, and
- Social and cultural background.

Among the above mentioned psychological factors, pain catastrophizing (the tendency to exaggerate a pain experience more than the average person and to feel more helpless about the pain) has been proven to be the most consistent and reliable predictor of the pain experience. Pain catastrophized thinking negatively affects pain experience and management by a person's tendency to focus on and exaggerate the threat of pain, while negatively evaluating his own ability to deal with the pain. Pain catastrophizing also negatively affects pain experience and management by increasing the risk of psychological distress, depression, and anxiety. Pain catastrophizing is also evidently linked to increased risk of disability.

Behavioral and psychosomatic medicines examine the complete risk profile of biological, psychological, and social factors associated with pain and develop a personalized treatment protocol to affect a behavioral change on the part of the patient and treat the pain, instead of just the biomedical aspect alone.

Unfortunately, psychosocial interventions for pain are mostly available only at tertiary care centers by highly trained health professionals, at considerable costs.

However, its principle is simple and everyone can apply it. All you need is knowledge and will power. For the knowledge, a great reference is Dr. John E. Sarno, MD's book *Healing Back Pain: The Mind-Body Connection*, published by Reed Business Information, Inc. 1999.

Most back pain sufferers are guilty of some degree of pain catastrophizing, fear of pain, and fear of movement. Stopping such behavior can help you significantly. Whether you get these mental behaviors out of your head on your own or with the assistance of a professional, the end result is similar. It is all in your head. Only you can get it out of your head, even with the specialized assistance.

You can do it. Just do it, now, today. You can always reach out to the specialized psychosocial intervention later on.

9. Aromatherapy

Aromatherapy is an ancient therapy and has been widely practiced in many cultures around the world. Aromatherapy uses various oils and extracts from vegetables, plants, and flowers to achieve a wide range of medicinal results.

Such oils and extracts have natural anti-spasmodic, anti-inflammatory and analgesic properties that can penetrate the skin and reach affected tissues within minutes, to help relieve pains in the back and other parts of the body.

A Polish study published in *Ortopedia Traumatologia Rehabilitacja* (Orthopedic Traumatology Rehabilitation) has shown that analgesic treatment with some vegetable aromatic oils was more effective than Ketoprofen (a known over-the-counter pain relief ingredient around the world).

A study published in *Complementary Therapies in Medicine* showed that Swedish massage with aromatic ginger oil led to significant improvements in pain intensity and disability, with both short and long-term effectiveness in treating chronic lower back pain for older adults. The study also showed that Swedish massage with aromatic ginger oil was more effective than traditional Thai massage without aromatic oil in reducing pain and improving disability at short and long-term assessments.

Another study published in *Complementary Therapies in Medicine* showed that eight-sessions of acupressure with aromatic lavender oil were an effective relief for short-term lower back pain. It effectively reduced pain intensity, improved walking time, and increased lateral spine flexion range (a range of motion of the spine while bending your back sideways).

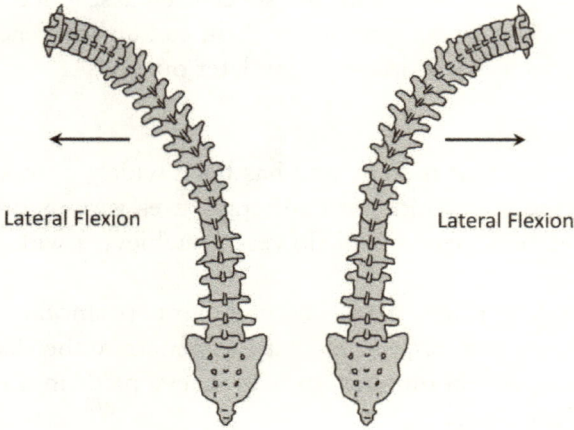

Source: Aaron Birch, Ryan Walsh, Diane Devita, Unique Mechanism of Chance Fracture in a Young Adult Male, WestJEM/ Department of Emergency Medicine, UC Irvine Health

Fig. 2.7

There are varieties of aroma oils that can be used for back pain relief. These oils can be used on their own or in a blend. The most effective application of aroma oil for back pain relief may be a blend of multiple oils. In a similar principle to oral medicines, in which effective ingredients are almost always mixed with a carrier ingredient, it is beneficial to mix an aroma oil or a blend of aroma oils with a carrier oil for better results.

If you wonder what aroma oils may be beneficial to your back, the following is a list of commonly used ones with their properties described:

- **Balsam Fir Essential Oil**: hypotensive, anti-rheumatic.
- **Chamomile Essential Oil**: anti-spasmodic, anti-inflammatory, analgesic, sedative, antiseptic, antibiotic, anti-depressant, and anti-infectious.
- **Clary Sage Essential Oil**: calming, anti-spasmodic, anti-inflammatory, antidepressant, and sedative.
- **Clove Essential Oil**: anti-septic, and anti-viral.
- **Copaiba Essential Oil (Copal)**: analgesic and anti-inflammation.
- **Cypress Essential Oil**: anti-spasmodic, anti-septic,

hemostatic, and sedative.

- **Elemi Essential Oil**: antiseptic, analgesic, and stimulative.
- **Frankincense Oil**: anti-inflammatory, antiseptic, disinfectant, and sedative.
- **Ginger Essential Oil**: anti-spasmodic, anti-inflammatory, and analgesic.
- **Helichrysum Essential Oil**: anti-spasmodic, anti-allergenic, anti-inflammatory, and anti-septic.
- **Lavender Essential Oil**: hypotensive, anti-inflammatory, analgesic, and blood circulation.
- **Marjoram Essential Oil**: analgesic, anti-spasmodic, antiseptic, antiviral, bactericidal, hypotensive, and sedative.
- **Myrrh Essential Oil**: anti-inflammatory, antispasmodic, and stimulative.
- **Peppermint Essential Oil**: anti-spasmodic and analgesic.
- **Rosemary Essential Oil**: analgesic
- **Thyme Essential Oil**: anti-spasmodic, anti-rheumatic, and antiseptic.
- **White Fir Essential Oil**: anti-rheumatic and anti-inflammatory.
- **Wintergreen Essential Oil**: analgesic, anti-rheumatic, anti-arthritic, anti-spasmodic, and antiseptic.
- **Yarrow Essential Oil**: anti-spasmodic, anti-inflammatory, anti-rheumatic, antiseptic, and hypotensive.

Similar to other natural remedies, aroma oils and extracts are less sensitive to dosage and seldom cause any undesirable side effects when used properly.

5

A Quick Roadmap For Beating Your Back Pain Fast

To get the right care to beat your back pain fast, first you must have a diagnosis.

How to Diagnose

There are two options to diagnose back pain – self-diagnosis and diagnosis by qualified healthcare professionals. Notice that "professionals" is a plural. In complicated cases, the causes are not easily identifiable, or in severe cases where highly invasive treatment may be required, or in a case of prolonged suffering, such as chronic pain, it is always a good idea to seek multiple healthcare professionals from various disciplines for solutions and recommendations.

Self-diagnosis and diagnosis by healthcare professionals often go hand in hand. Self-diagnosis often precedes visits to professionals. Self-diagnosis helps you get the right help faster.

For example, after falling from your mountain bike, if you heard a cracking sound in your back and feel instant and severe pain in your back, you may want to go or be taken directly to a hospital because you may have a spinal fracture. You may visit your family doctor if your back pain is accompanied by pain, malfunction or discomfort with any of your internal organ. Or you may visit a massage therapist for back pain relief if your back pain is accompanied by stiffness or spasm in your back.

If you have suffered back pain for years, and you have ruled out any cause outside of your back, you may wish to seek help from a chiropractic doctor or an osteopathic doctor. Take an active role in getting the right help faster. This will save you valuable time, and keep the window of opportunity open for you to get the care you need, and avoid unnecessary suffering.

Diagnosis by qualified professionals can legally only be done by professionals who are authorized to diagnose you due to their special training. Not every healthcare professional is authorized to diagnose you.

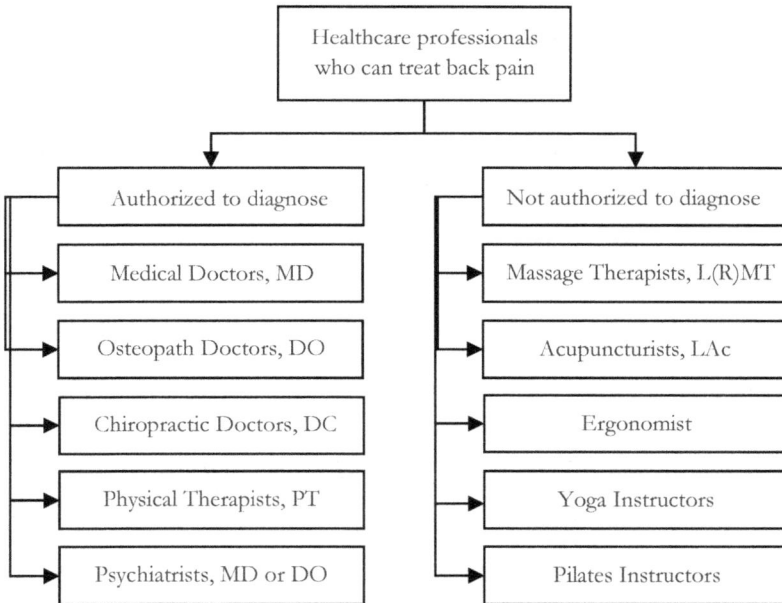

Source: compiled by Patrick Lee

Fig. 2.8

If the cause of your back pain is not completely clear, seek one of the professionals who is authorized to diagnose it.

Obviously not all authorized diagnosticians are spine or back specialists. Some are far more knowledgeable about the spine and the back than others, due to their medical training and the nature of their medical practice.

Generally speaking, osteopathic and chiropractic doctors have dramatically more medical training, practical experience, and skills with the human spine and back disorders than any of their other medical peers from other disciplines. For example, a family doctor may devote 5 to 10 percent of their professional time and attention to the treatment of back pain, while an osteopathic or chiropractic doctor may devote 50 to 100 percent of their professional time and attention to spine and back disorders.

From a basic medical training point of view, the total number of training hours a medical graduate receives from their school may vary dramatically. The training they receive on the musculoskeletal system is critical because, to many doctors especially family doctors, the training they received during their school years is the only training they have on the musculoskeletal system.

Osteopathic studies include 300-hours of training in hands-on manual treatments and the on musculoskeletal system, according to the Osteopathic Medical College Information Book 2010. In the USA, their education is virtually identical to those of general medical doctors, however, with an additional 200-hours of Osteopathic Manipulative Medicine (OMM).

For chiropractic doctors in the States, about 550-hours are devoted to learning about spinal anatomy, biomechanics, adjustive techniques, analysis, and diagnostics in colleges of chiropractic, as a part of a complete curriculum of 4,200-hours of classroom, laboratory, and clinical experience.

With general medical doctors, such as family doctors, the situation is very different. In a 2003 survey by the Bone and Joint Decade in 32 countries (K. Dreinhöfer, personal communication, 2003), the median total teaching time on the musculoskeletal system received by a medical school graduate was only:

- 97-hours on orthopaedics,
- 30-hours of lectures and courses,
- 21-hours on trauma surgery,
- 26-hours on rheumatology,
- And 20-hours on physical medicine rehabilitation.

Considering that the average length of an undergraduate medical education is six years and at many of these schools these courses are not obligatory, this shows a significant shortcoming in doctors' training in musculoskeletal issues.

In the case of physiotherapists, training hours on the musculoskeletal system varies dramatically. However, according to the curriculum of Georgia State University, the total number of training hours on musculoskeletal system for a physiotherapy graduate is about 20 to 30-hours.

Total Hours of Formal Training on Musculoskeletal

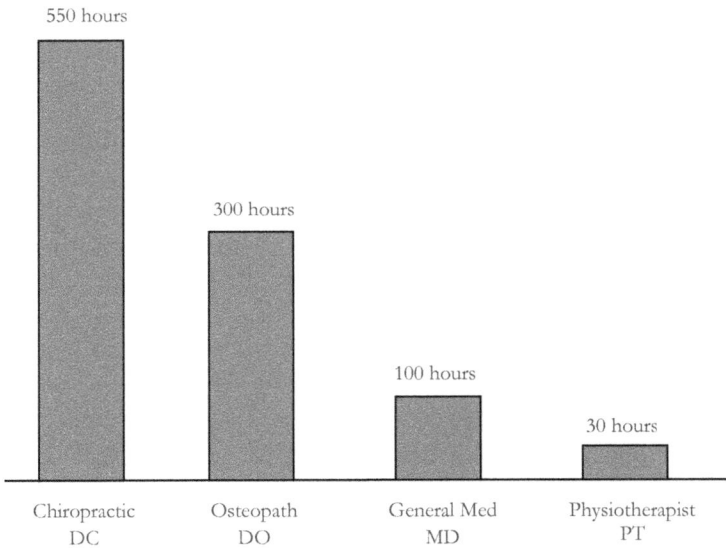

Source: compiled by Patrick Lee

Fig. 2.9

The above chart should not give you the idea that chiropractic medicine should be the first care to seek for all back pain. For those that are caused by musculoskeletal problems, chiropractic is indeed a good choice of first care. However, if your back pain is caused by problems with inner organs, the wise choice is an osteopathic doctor or a conventional medical doctor, such as your family doctor. The following section offers details on how to chose the suitable first care type for your condition.

What Type of Care to Start With First?

There are many ways to analyze your situation to determine what care may be most suitable to you as the first point of consultation.

For example, you may start with any existing diagnosis you may already have, or you may start with the fact that your pain is acute or chronic, or you may start with whether or not your pain had a quick onset. For practical reasons, we have chosen to start with whether your back pain is due to a severe physical trauma or accident, because the answer to this question may require you to get to the emergency room of a hospital as fast as possible. Not that you would have the time to read a book when you have had a trauma or been in an accident and are experiencing severe back. But this situation only accounts for a small minority of the total back pain instances each year.

The next important factor in your self-assessment is to know whether your pain started with an awkward bending, twisting, lifting, and other seemingly trivial physical movement or activity.

Sometimes the movement may not be awkward at all, for example, say you bent down to pick up a pencil on the floor, or while you lifted a grocery bag out of the car's trunk. Sudden back pain may immobilize you. If your back pain started with an awkward or not so awkward bending, twisting, lifting, or other trivial movement, your best bet may be visiting a chiropractic clinic. A large portion of back pains belong to this category. But for further analysis, you may wish to follow the road map in section 11 of this book. We will discuss more on this on the following pages.

If, however, your back pain is not caused by a severe trauma, accident or a trivial movement, you need to assess carefully other aspects of your health condition. If you have had back surgery in the past, then you need to go back to the hospital or your surgeon to find out if your operation is failing. Over time many surgical operations may fail, especially when an implant is involved. Even though the metal implants or screws may seem to be strong, they can't withstand the continued repetitive stresses placed on them by the movement of your spine, and may eventually become fatigued, loose, or even broken.

You are aware that the stress placed on the surgical metals in your spine can be significant enough to break the hard metal. Imagine what this stress could do to your vertebrae, discs, ligaments, and the muscles of your spine. Yes, you are right, the stress can hurt them too. And there is a condition called Repetitive Strain Injury. Prolonged improper use of your back or spine can lead to devastating consequences to your back. In fact, repetitive strain injuries are a leading cause for back pain. Slouching at your computer desk or on your couch watching TV are among the most frequent causes leading to repetitive strain injury. More on this later.

Many medical conditions may lead to back pain, such as cancer, kidney problems, ovary problems, bleeding or infection inside the pelvis, or an aortic aneurysm. Conventional medicine is the most suitable first point of consultation for such cases. However, it is important to realize that back pain is rarely caused by such serious conditions. According to the University of Iowa, in a study of 1,200 patients with acute back pain, less than 1 percent of patients with back pain had a serious condition including a fracture, infection, cancer, or multiple nerve root compressions.

Conditions, such as infection of cartilage and vertebra, arthritis, and Paget's Disease, may cause considerable pain. Again, conventional medicine, such as a specialist or your family doctor should serve as your first point of consultation.

Other less severe conditions, such as shingles may cause back pain. If your back pain is accompanied by a fever, it may indicate a more serious health issue. Body temperature is a reflection of the body's fight against infections, virus, and enemy cells. If these causes are strong enough to cause both fever and back pain, you need to see your doctor of conventional medicine as soon as possible.

Do you have scoliosis or an abnormal pregnancy? Some degree of back pain in such situations is rather normal. You may wish to see a chiropractic clinic, a manual osteopath clinic, or a massage clinic for help. And you most likely will be happy to find out that the treatments you receive will work well for you.

Your Quick Roadmap for Your First Care

The following chart is a simplified roadmap to help you find the right type of care to consult first to save you time, money, and suffering.

Right care depends on the cause of your condition. Needless to say, your back will have its speedy recovery by seeking the right care for its particular condition, not by simply seeking a care. Mismatch of care and your condition will only result in:

- Your prolonged suffering,

Applicable Care By Causes Of Back Pain	
1. in the back	symptoms: pure pain, mobility issues, pain in upper, middle, lower back, pain may radiate to legs
major trauma	hospital
minor trauma	chiropractic; osteopath
poor posture	chiropractic; osteopath, physical therapy
inflammation	family doctor; specialist, hospital
degeneration	chiropractic; osteopath, hospital
chronic	chiropractic; osteopath, physical therapy, massage, acupuncture, Pilates, Alexander tech, Yoga, Taichi,
abnormal spine	chiropractic; osteopath, hospital
cause unclear	chiropractic, osteopath, physical therapy, massage, acupuncture, Pilates, specialist, hospital
2. in the pelvis	symptoms: pain with other symptoms such as pelvic obliquity, hip contracture, scoliosis, pain in lower or mid back
	chiropractic, osteopath, hospital
3. in legs/feet	symptoms: pain with other symptoms such as leg length discrepancy, pelvic obliquity, pain in lower or mid back
	chiropractic, osteopath, podiatry
4. inside the body	symptoms: pain with other symptoms such as fever, weight loss, pain in lower back
	Family doctor, specialist, hospital
5. in the mind	symptoms: pain constant, depression, relationship problems, family issues, workplace stress, pain in lower or upper back
	helpful books, positive friends, pets, nature, psychiatrist, hypnotherapy

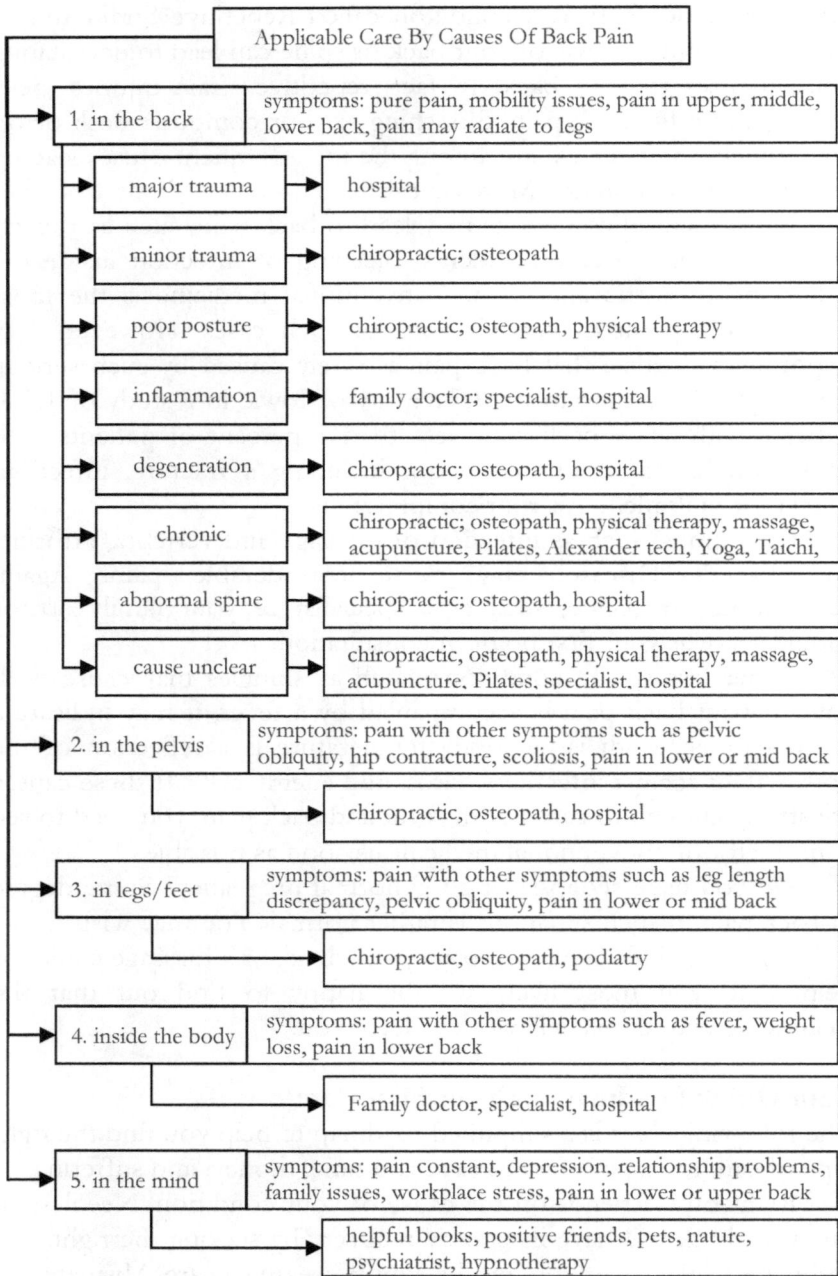

Source: compiled by Patrick Lee

Fig. 2.10

- Dissatisfaction with your care giver,
- Wasting of money,
- A missed window of opportunity to heal,
- The worsening of your condition,
- Even suffering perpetually with a belief that your problem can't be resolved.

By no means is this road map perfect. It doesn't work for all sufferers all the time. However, it does serve as a practical starting point and may help save you up to 80 percent of your time while on your journey of searching for the relief that your back deserves.

The most important question to ask when determining what care is the most suitable for you to seek first is: where does the cause of your back pain lie? Is it in your back, your pelvis, your lower extremities, your body or your mind?

1. If you experience difficulties with range of motion, and your pain is not accompanied by any complicating symptoms, such as fever and weight loss, or any abnormality in your pelvis, legs or feet, the cause may be in your back itself. Maybe a trauma happened to your back, an inflammation in your muscles or joints, an injury to the muscles, tendons, ligaments, discs or vertebrae.

a. If your pain started after a major trauma, such as a car accident, a fall from a high position, and you suspect that you may have suffered bone damage, you need to go straight to a hospital. Don't wait. Don't think you should seek your family doctor, and any other doctors first, then go to hospital, because your family doctor or any other health care professional could do very little to a situation involving bone damage.

b. If your pain started after a minor trauma such as the wrong movement of your body, by lifting a garbage bin, you may want to go and see a chiropractic doctor, manual osteopath doctor, a massage therapist, or an acupuncturist.

c. If your pain is due to poor posture, such as Forward Head Posture, a hunched back, or slouching while sitting, you may want to see a chiropractor, a manual osteopathic doctor, an ergonomist, or a physiotherapist, to help you correct your posture and reset your proper spinal alignment.

d. If your pain is due to an inflammation, such as arthritis, you may want to see your family doctor for a referral to a specialist.

e. If your pain is chronic or unknown in nature for which your family doctor and a conventional medical specialist have helped you rule out any cause linked to any of your inner organs, your best bet is to seek help from the manual therapies, such as chiropractic, osteopath, physiotherapy, massage therapy, acupuncture, Pilates, Yoga, Alexander technique, Feldnkreis technique, Taichi, and so on.

f. If your pain is due to a muscle imbalance, your best choice may be chiropractic, physiotherapy, Pilates, Yoga, Alexander technique, Feldnkreis technique, and Taichi.

2. If you have back pain and also abnormality in your pelvis, such as pelvis obliquity and ischial tuberosity obliquity, you may want to pay close attention to these conditions to see if your back pain is actually caused by these issues. If the cause of your pain is not identified by looking elsewhere, attention needs to be paid to these issues too. A good starting point for this is to visit a chiropractor or a manual osteopathic doctor.

3. If you have some structural or habitual abnormality in your legs or feet, you need to pay close attention to these issues to see their relevance to your back pain. These issues may include leg length discrepancy, hyperpronation or hypersupination of foot. Shoes with unevenly worn heels or unleveled standing or sitting platform would also lead to tilted spine and increased stress and tension in the back that, over time, could cause pain in the back.

Indeed, the musculoskeletal system of our body is an interconnected chain of elements from toe to head. Any abnormality with an element at a lower level may affect the wellbeing of the elements above.

To closely keep in mind the relevance of our legs and feet to our back, it is good to remember the song "Dem Bone" by James Weldon Johnson:

"...Toe bone connected to the foot bone,
Foot bone connected to the heel bone,
Heel bone connected to the ankle bone,
Ankle bone connected to the shin bone,
Shin bone connected to the knee bone,

Knee bone connected to the thigh bone,
Thigh bone connected to the hip bone,
Hip bone connected to the back bone,
Back bone connected to the shoulder bone,
Shoulder bone connected to the neck bone,
Neck bone connected to the head bone..."

4. If your pain is accompanied by complicating symptoms, such as: a fever, weight loss, general fatigue or pain in your abdomen, bowel problems, or urinary problems, chances are that the cause of your back pain is in your body. There may be issues with your inner organs. They can be as harmless as a strong period, or as serious as pelvis infection, kidney problems, even cancer. You should visit your family doctor or a hospital as soon as possible.

5. If your pain is chronic or regular, and you suffer from relationship issues, mental or emotional stress, or even depression, chances are that a big part of the cause of your back pain is in your mind. In such cases, your best bet will be to read some helpful books, increase your socialization with positive friends, distance yourself from the source of the emotional or mental stress. You may also want to seek help from a clinical psychiatry or psychology professionals who specializes in back pain related issues.

Of course, back pain is a complex issue. In most cases, diagnostics professionals need special expertise and a concerted multi-disciplinary effort. The above framework is an overly simplified approach to help you quickly determine what care would be the most suitable one to start with. Once you have begun this journey, the initial care professional, especially diagnosticians, such as a conventional medical doctor, chiropractic doctor, osteopathic doctor, or physiotherapist, will help you with detailed diagnostics, and may refer you to other disciplines of care as your particular details may require.

Going to the right diagnostician at the very beginning is critical to the speedy recovery of your back or spinal problems. To most people, the above simple road map will help you save tons of time, money, and suffering.

Always keep the following two points in mind. First, the fact that one particular care giver's treatment didn't work out for you, doesn't indicate that his or her discipline of care is not suitable to you. Second, the fact that a few care givers or disciplines of care have not been able to help you doesn't mean that your condition can't be helped.

In today's world, chances are that there already exists a suitable treatment to your particular condition, that can help you relieve your suffering, somewhere. You may have had or observed such an experience from your family, friends, co-workers, neighbors, or fellow members of social or professional clubs, where someone who had a condition that was pronounced by a certain care giver as untreatable and hopeless, but had found the right care for his or her health problem. Back pain is not different in this regard. The continued effort of searching for the right care is the key for your relief and recovery. It is not a false hope. It is a reality.

If, and only if, you want to read more, to be able to get more control over your condition, the following are some further details you may find interesting, helpful, and beneficial. Again, please note that they are still over-simplified. They are not designed to help you diagnose. Instead, they are only designed to provide you with a little more detail on the various potential situations.

If the Pain is in Your Lower Back
One of the first questions you want to ask yourself in this case is whether your pain shoots down your legs. If so, a nerve that is inside, or is exiting your lumbar spine may have been pinched. If you do not have severe disc or vertebral degeneration or damage, your best bet is to see a chiropractic doctor or a manual osteopath first, because they are very effective in helping you realign your spine and reducing nerve interference in the spine.

Is your pain in one of your buttocks and the back of the thigh beneath it? If so you may have:
- Sacroiliac strain (often caused by a combination of vertical compression and rapid rotation of the butt, or by a backwards fall on the ground),
- Gluteus medius dysfunction (the weakening of the gluteus medius, often experienced by runners and joggers. Weakened glutes medius on one leg often cause the hip the drop at the oposit side when standing on the

said leg. This could lead to the abnormal stress even strain in the stabilizing muscles in the lower back, over time, causing pain in lower back.),

- Piriformis syndrome (a condition in which the piriformis muscle spasms and causes buttock pain. The piriformis muscle can also irritate the nearby sciatic nerve and cause sciatic pain, numbness and tingling), or
- Inflammation.

You may wish to visit a chiropractic or a manual osteopath clinic. If your pain does not reduce, you could visit a conventional medical doctor, just in case you may have any inflammation or any other unexpected issues.

Is your pain mainly in the hip, groin or on the front of your thigh? This may be an indication of a hip joint problem or osteoarthritis. See your family doctor for a referral to a specialist.

Does your pain get worse when standing or sitting for a prolonged period? Your pain may be postural pain or caused by facet joint compression. See a chiropractic or manual osteopath doctor first.

Is your pain accompanied by the locking of your back in one position? This may be an indication of your lumbar instability or hypermobility of your lumbar spine. As a natural self-protective mechanism, your back will lock down to prevent any damage that may be caused by the instability of your lumbar spine. See a chiropractic doctor, a manual osteopathic doctor, a physiotherapist, or an exercise expert who can help strengthen your core and lumbar area, such as a Pilates, Feldenkrais method, Alexander technique, and Yoga instructor.

Does your back pain get worse when you bend or twist your back, when you lift something, or after a sleep? This may indicate a disc protrusion, or postural pain. Visit a chiropractor, or a manual osteopath for your initial consultation.

Is your back pain accompanied by pain in both of your legs that worsens with prolonged standing or walking? If so, one of your vertebrae may have been displaced forward causing your nerve to be pinched. Or you may have a spinal stenosis (the narrowing of your spinal canal) that may have started to interfere with your spinal cord or nerve roots. Such a situation can be easily clarified by an X-ray image. In most cases, you want to visit a chiropractor or manual osteopath first. They will provide effective care for you, if your condition is mild enough. If your condition is too advanced, they will advise you to see a conventional medical specialist, such as an orthopedic surgeon.

If the Pain is in Your Neck

The neck is the most vulnerable part of the spine. Pain in the neck may indicate something more serious than you would think.

Is the pain in your neck accompanied by a stiff neck, nausea, headache, vomiting, drowsiness, or confusion? If so, you may have inflammation in the membranes that covers the brain and the spinal cord. Or there may be internal bleeding in your brain (a brain hemorrhage). Go and visit a hospital or your family doctor for a referral as fast as possible. In such a situation, time is valuable, it is literally your life!

Do you experience difficulty in controlling your arms and legs, or experience weaknesses in your limbs? It may be an indication of a spinal cord injury. Again, go and visit a hospital or a spinal specialist, as quickly as possible.

Has your pain been progressing and is accompanied by intermittent numbness or a tingling in your hands? This may be an indication of osteoarthritis. In such an event, manual treatment often could only relieve the symptoms and would not be able to treat the cause. Your best bet may be conventional medical professionals. However, if you find the treatment by conventional medicine too intrusive or risky, and that your pain is manageable, you may wish to seek manual treatments, such as a chiropractic doctor, manual osteopath, physiotherapy, massage therapy, yoga, Pilate's, Feldenkrais method, and/or the Alexander technique.

Is your pain confined to the neck, and characterized by a quick onset within a few hours? It may be due to whiplash. Most whiplash does not involve vertebral damage or soft tissue tear. In such situations, you may want to start by visiting a chiropractor or a manual osteopath. If however, you suspect any vertebral damage or soft tissue damage may be involved, then you may want to visit a hospital or a conventional medical specialist first.

Is your pain accompanied by numbness, or tingling that extends down your arm? It may be an indication of disc protrusion in the neck. In most situations, you may want to visit a chiropractic or manual osteopath first. However, in the minority cases where the disc protrusion can't be successfully treated by manual treatments, your only remaining option may then be conventional medicine, whose treatment may be highly intrusive, such as surgery.

Does your pain shoot down the shoulders and the upper arms that are exaggerated by even minor movements in and around the neck? This may indicate a disc protrusion that interferes with the nerves in the neck, or a facet joint strain in the neck. This situation is similar to the situation above, where you want to see a chiropractic or manual osteopath first. If relief by such treatment is not satisfactory, your disc or facet problem may be too advanced. You may wish to consult a conventional medical specialist for the spine or the back.

Is your neck extra painful and stiff when waking up? It may be a sign of damage to the neck muscles or blood supply caused by poor sleeping posture, or previous physical activity. You could consider visiting a massage therapist, physiotherapist, a chiropractic, or manual osteopath doctor.

Is your present pain the result of previous acute pain? Your pain may be a secondary pain caused by your body's self-protective mechanism. You may want to see a massage therapist, a physiotherapist, a chiropractor, or a manual osteopath doctor.

Does your pain worsen after being in one position, such as working on a computer or reading a book, for a prolonged period? This may be an indication of disc protrusion or muscle tension. Consider seeing a massage therapist, a chiropractic doctor, or a manual osteopath doctor for first consultation and treatment.

If the Pain is in Your Mid Back

Due to the presence of rib cages, the mid back is better protected than the lower back and the neck. The mid back is less prone to injury because it is not responsible for the bending, twisting, and turning of the body. However, occasionally it also becomes injured or painful.

Is your pain in the mid back and radiating around your rib cage? Does breathing cause sharp pain in your mid back? Was it due to a physical trauma to your back? If so, you may be suffering a broken rib or severe spinal injury. Visit a hospital or a conventional medical specialist.

Did your pain that radiates around your rib cage start with a trivial movement? You may be suffering from degenerative fracture, pleurisy (inflammation of the membrane around your lungs), bronchitis, or pneumonia. Visit a hospital or a conventional medical doctor.

If your answers are no to all the above questions, the cause may be a certain degree of disc protrusion. See a chiropractic or manual osteopath for initial consultation.

If your pain does not radiate around, but progresses steadily, and is accompanied by general fatigue, it may be tissue inflammation (abscess) or even a tumor. Visit your family doctor or a specialist of conventional medicine. A manual care giver may not be able to help you much.

Is your pain relieved by a change of body position or a gentle movement? It may be postural pain. See a chiropractor or a manual osteopath for postural correction or improvement, or see a massage therapist for tension relief. You may also use exercise therapies, such as Pilate's, Yoga, the Feldenkrais method, or the Alexander technique.

Does your pain follow intensive physical activities? If so, it may be a muscular problem, because the mid back is a center for back muscles, especially those that control the movement of the upper body and the upper extremities. Even minor damage to any of these muscles can cause pain in the mid back. See a physiotherapist or a massage therapist for rehab. A chiropractor or a manual osteopath may be helpful too.

Did your pain start with a physical trauma or a trivial movement to your back, and worsen with body movement? If so, you may suffer from damage to your spinal cord, a degenerative fracture, and other medical conditions that are best dealt with by conventional medical doctors or specialists. Go and see them as your first choice.

If your condition is not covered by the above questions or scenarios, your option would be evenly spread out among conventional medicine, chiropractic doctors, manual osteopaths, and physiotherapy.

6

4 Secrets to Help You Avoid the Wrong Caregivers

In determining the right solution to go with, the DON'Ts are as critical as the DO's. Avoiding the wrong caregiver is critical. This applies to all disciplines of care, from chiropractic to psychosomatic medicine. The reason is simple, while most care givers are competent and professional enough to put your interests above their own, some may, from time to time, not be sufficiently competent, or not professional enough to put their own interest above yours.

The following are some DON'Ts:

1. Don't go with a caregiver, if you hear the person say that his or her treatment, program, technique, or product can treat your back pain regardless.

    The truth is that back pain is a complicated matter. There is simply no one solution that can cure all back pain. Ask the potential provider, what the limitations of his or her treatment, program, technique, or product are. If someone tells you that his or her solution has no limitation, he or she either doesn't know what he or she is talking about, or is simply lying to you. Either reason should be sufficient for you to stay away from this potential provider. And there are an abundance of both cases in the real world.

The provider who truly can't tell you the limitations of their solution are often new to the art of healing and don't know the limitation of their art or their individual competence. Such situations may happen with new healthcare graduates, or with a professional new to a certain technique or product.

True experts know the shortcomings of their treatment, program, and product far more than any third-party. A true expert will not hesitate to discuss the shortcomings of his or her solutions, partly because they are, while acutely aware of the shortcomings of their solution, are also fully confident of the strengths, benefits, and advantages of his or her solution.

2. Don't go with a caregiver, if you hear the person globally put down other care, programs, techniques or products in order to boost his or her own offering. The reality is that each care, treatment, program, technique or product has its own relative advantages, strengths, and unique set of benefits.

Globally putting down others shows a lack of knowledge or ethics on the part of the person who puts down others. Run as soon as you sense someone's lack of professional ethics. A service provider who is not ethical to his or her peers would hardly be ethical to you. What such people are mostly interested in tends to be your wallet instead of your wellbeing. Due to high economic pressures, unfortunately there are way too many of these providers of many services and in all fields.

3. Don't go with a caregiver, if he or she rambles on-and-on with vague stories about miracle treatments, medicines or devices. Or if all you hear about is this miracle treatment's name more than three times without hearing any details about what that miracle solution really is, how it really works or any other verifiable and measurable results.

These are the typical precursors of high pressure sales tactics of mediocre solutions. You don't need to waste your time on any bit of it.

Providers with truly outstanding solutions will almost immediately show you the measureable results that their offering has achieved, such as through third-party clinical study results, peer reviews, testimonials or on credible third-party public forums. They will all be eager to tell you what their solution really is, and why their solution may work so well for you.

4. Don't go with a caregiver, if you hear from the person that you have to put up with the problem for the rest of your life.

   As complicated and difficult as it may be to treat back pain, there is always a way to reduce, relieve, contain, manage, and even eliminate it.

   The fact that someone tells you that you have to live with your back pain, often only indicates that their expertise or knowledge has hit the wall. There are many others, with more experience or a deeper knowledge within the same discipline, who can help. There are many more clinical approaches and techniques in that same discipline, that can help. There are also many medical disciplines beyond that particular discipline, that may offer hope and a tangible result.

   The fact that someone would say you have no hope often only represents the opinion of that one person, within one particular technique or approach, within one particular discipline. Go out and talk to more potential solution providers.

A doctor is not a doctor, just like a carpenter is not a carpenter and the color gray is not the color gray. When we deal with simpler terms of reference, we have common sense and a healthy skepticism. We may disagree or argue with them about what they say. Unfortunately, when it comes to more sophisticated terms of reference, such as healthcare to our back, we often take what a healthcare provider says as an indisputable truth.

The truth is that a doctor is a doctor because he or she has obtained a medical license. And in order to obtain that license, a doctor must take an exam. Do you think that all doctors get 100 percent on their medical exams in order to get their license? No. Depending on the discipline, often a 60 percent grade is all that is required, which means 40 percent of their knowledge mastery is incorrect. This may translate 40 percent mistakes in their diagnoses and treatment. While exam scores do not always directly translate into the effectiveness of their treatments for their patients, this is an indication that most doctors are not the perfect doctors. They have shortcomings and make mistakes just like anyone else does.

While respecting the advice of your health care providers, take their advice with a healthy grain of salt. A truly perfect doctor or therapist will tend to see the world as filled with promises and possibilities. The possibility of you having to live with your pain for the rest of your life would rarely be the possibility they see for you.

7

8 Things You Can Do To Minimize The Risk Of Misdiagnosis

According to Jerome Groopman, Professor of Medicine at Harvard University, misdiagnosis happens in 20 percent of medical cases. Misdiagnoses often leads to:

- Prolonged suffering,
- A waste of money,
- Increased agony,
- Decreased satisfaction with the care received,
- And more serious consequences such as the reversible loss of opportunity to recover.

You must do everything possible to stay out of the statistics of misdiagnosed cases.

But could you reduce the risk of the misdiagnosis? Here are eight initiatives you can take:

1. **Prepare for your meeting with your doctor.** Doctors often make their diagnoses about your situation in 18-seconds. Rambling on about your situation could only lead to an increased risk of

misdiagnosis. Make a list of facts about your condition that answers the five W's and the one H (who, what, where, when, why and how). You also should add to that list "how much," how much pain you are in. Make sure you tell your doctor when, where, and how your symptoms or problem began, and what was going on with your body when you first begin to feel the symptom or problem. And make sure you tell your doctor the stages of progression of your problem, and what was going on with your body when the stage transitions happened.

2. **Tell the full and factual story about your condition.** Do not tell irrelevant stories. Do not interpret your condition for your doctor. Telling irrelevant stories will only waste time, raise mental blocks with your doctor, and increase the risk of misdiagnosis. Tell your doctor nothing but the facts. Make sure you answer his or her questions closely, instead of going on for wide circles, never hitting the center – or important information. Keep the fluff to a minimum. Actively offer additional facts if your doctor didn't ask, but you feel it is important for him or her to know.

3. **Ask your doctor point blank what his or her diagnosis of your problem is, and then ask him or her to explain the typical symptoms of this diagnosis.** Listen carefully to see if those typical symptoms match those of yours. Don't simply let go if your doctor says "the typical symptoms of your diagnosis are exactly the same as those of yours." If the typical symptoms described don't match those you are currently going through, you need to let your doctor know. "That symptom doesn't really match mine. I actually feel this way _____ (fill in the blank)."

4. **Help your doctor double check his/her diagnosis by asking questions.** Ask questions such as: "what other factors could be at play?" "What else do you think could it possibly be to cause my problem?" "Could I have more than one thing wrong with me?"

5. **Voice your concerns and ask your doctor to repeat a test or an imaging scan, if the result is too surprising to be true.** Mistakes happen with tests and medical imaging. "I've seen lab mistakes dozens of times," says Robert Wachter, Chief of the

Division of Hospital Medicine at the University of California, San Francisco Medical Center. According to an investigation by US News, failure rates of medical tests and imaging can be as high as three to five percent, which means that one out of every 20 to 30 results could be wrong. Your results may be one of them. Your results could have been mixed up with another patient's. Your test samples could have been contaminated.

In most cases, your doctor will be glad to repeat a test or an imaging scan (such as an MRI, or an X-ray) for you, if you tell him/her about your concern or the abnormality of your test results. Especially if the results serve as a basis for an invasive treatment such as surgery.

6.   **Make sure you are on time for your appointment.** Doctors are busy. He or she will risk being late for subsequent appointments, if you are late for yours. Late arrival of a patient will put the doctor under more time pressure. And time pressure and rush are the key causes for mistakes that you don't want.

7.   **Make sure you have a cordial relationship with your doctor.** If you don't feel you have the right chemistry with your doctor, he or she will feel likewise. Lack of constructive chemistry will increase the risk of overlooking or misunderstanding some symptoms or clues, which in turn, raises the risk of an incorrect diagnosis. Work on improving the relationship or seek out another doctor, if you can.

8.   **No diagnosis is better than misdiagnosis or inaccurate diagnosis.** Reasons for spinal problems or back pains are often not easily known or immediately diagnosable. If a doctor says that he or she is not sure about the cause of the problem, you need to respect his or her honest answer. You could explore with your doctor the next steps and how to move closer towards a reasonable diagnosis. You could ask your doctor if another medicine discipline could help reach a diagnosis. Or you can seek further opinions on your own initiative. Don't pressure your doctor for a diagnosis, because it could only lead to an inaccurate diagnosis.

8

30 Questions You Must Ask Your Doctors

It is critical for you to become a partner to your doctor, in order to recover fast and stay well longer. One of the important things to do towards this pursuit is to ask the right questions when seeing your doctor.

Here are some specific categories of questions, along with the questions you need to ask your doctors, to turn your angry back into a smiling back.

Questions you should ask your doctor to help find the true cause of your problem:

- What is your diagnosis of my problem?

- What are the typical symptoms of this diagnosis? And why?

- That symptom doesn't really match mine. I actually feel this way _____ (fill in the blank). What could cause this symptom that I feel?

- Is the cause of my back pain in my back or inside my body? And why?

- Is my problem due to an injury, infection, inflammation, musculoskeletal imbalance, physical stress, mental stress, problems with my inner organs, or any other reason? And why?

- What other factors could be at play?

- What else do you think could it possibly be causing my problem?

- Could I have more than one thing wrong with me?

- What could be the secondary cause for my back problem? And why?

- Why doesn't my back pain go away after such a long time?

- How come my body hasn't healed itself this time?

Questions you should ask your doctor to help reach the right choice of treatment:

- Does this treatment you suggest, deal with my symptoms or the underlying cause?

- How long does the effect of this treatment last?

- Do I need to repeat this treatment? If so, how often?

- What treats the cause instead of just the symptoms of my problem?

- What treatment offers a sustainable resolution to my issues?

- Does this treatment address the primary cause or the secondary cause?

- What less invasive treatment could be applied for my condition?

- Are there natural and effective solutions to my problem?

- What other medical disciplines do you recommend I seek for a second opinion?

- What questions do I need to ask when I see them?

Questions you can ask your doctor to stay well for the longer term:

- What should I do to prolong the effects of the treatment?

- What can I do to prevent my problem from repeating?

- Are there any lifestyle changes I need to make?

- Are there any solutions that can help me in my daily life?

- What do I need to do differently in my life from now on?

- How can I take on more responsibility for my health?

- How is stress affecting my health and life?

- What can I do to reduce or eliminate my stress?

- How can I improve my lifestyle choices?

PART THREE
THE SECRET OF YOUR BACK
- WHAT KEEPS IT HAPPY

Read this chapter, if you want to maintain your spinal health, or prevent back pain from happening or recurring, or to slow down spinal degeneration.

1

7 Secret Body Habits You Must Build

Back pain not only is pervasive but also tends to reoccur. Prevention is possible and critical.

Since most back pain is caused by trivial matters, it is critical to pay attention to the "trivial" matters. Such matters include maintaining a good posture especially when you sit and sleep, using your body in the right way. In other words:

- Applying the right body mechanics to your daily activities at work and at home,
- Exercising and strengthening your back and core muscles,
- Eating the right foods and taking in the right nutrition,
- Maintaining a healthy body weight,
- Wearing the right shoes (hint not high heels, ladies),
- Using the right dynamic or adaptive ergonomics at work and at home, including using the right seats and chairs, the right tools, and last but not least,

- The right assistive devices, such as neck, back and buttock supports, shoe insoles and so on.

If early symptoms were addressed properly and preventative measures were taken, 95 percent of herniated disc patients would NOT require surgery.

Most back pains are due to poor body biomechanics or overuse. And overuse is often the result of poor body mechanics. Many dancers tilt their pelvis forward when lifting their female partner. Such a tilt leads to a hyper lordosis (abnormally deep curve in lower back) that significantly worsens the biomechanics in the lower lumbar spine. Over time, such actions often lead to lower back pain for dancers.

Using your body the right way in most activities is not easy. However, making the right way a habit will make things a lot easier for you. Use your back as sensible as you use your teeth. Use your body correctly both in your professional and private life.

1. Keep Motion in Your Back, Even When Sitting

The human body is not built for sitting. Physical vitality is in the movement, not in the stillness. You need to keep motion in your back as much as you can when you are awake, even while sitting. Actually sitting is one of the leading causes for back pain. Sedentary office workers, taxi drivers, truck drivers, public transit drivers, and pilots are among those who are most susceptive to back pain, due to their frequent prolonged sitting still.

It is the nature of the human body, that as soon as you sit still for more than 20-minutes, the deep stabilizing muscles in your lower back start to tense and stiffen, which often leads to stiffness, pain or fatigue in your lower back. To prevent such back pain caused by sitting, static ergonomic supports are not sufficient. You must prevent your deep stabilizing muscles from tensing to the extent you can. To achieve this objective, you either need to get up from your seat every 20-minutes or use a seat with a dynamic seating foundation, such as the SambaRX stability seat or the Back Vitalizer multifunctional dynamic seat.

Physical inactivity is one of the controllable habits that cause six out of 10 deaths in Ontario, Canada. And for most people in today's society, sitting is the most prevalent cause for physical inactivity.

While trying to maintain a good sitting posture, it is important to keep motion in your back while sitting, by getting up and moving around, or by incorporating a dynamic seating foundation or applying a dynamic back support that can accommodate or even encourage the movement in your back.

Take breaks frequently. If you work in front of a computer and often forget about taking the necessary break while sitting, use some ways to remind you of the breaks. You can set your cell phone for regular reminders. You can set your computer for regular reminders. You can even put a big bottle of water on your desk and drink it frequently and let your bladder remind and force you to get up and take breaks from your sitting, or simply get a dynamic seating device that can help keep the motion in your back continuously while you sit.

2. Keep the Right Curvature in the Back

Keeping a healthy curvature in your lower back can make your spine 150 percent stronger.

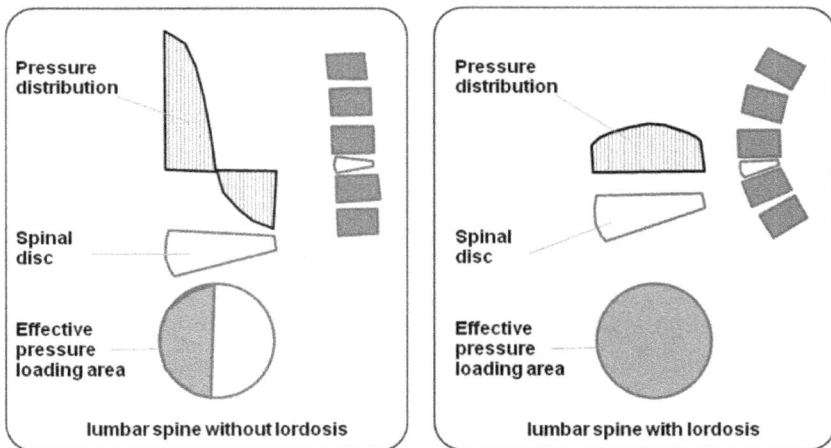

Source: compiled by Patrick Lee

Fig. 3.1

Our spine is not built to be flat. When the lumbar spine flattens, the loading pressure on the spinal discs shifts towards the anterior edge of the disc, which is especially true for adults due to the gradual degeneration of the spinal discs. While the size of the effective pressure loading area reduces, the pressure itself peaks. With a flattened lumbar spine, the effective pressure loading area on the corresponding spinal discs could be reduced by up to 60 percent, which increases the peak pressure around the anterior edge of the spinal disc often by more than 150 percent. As a result, the weight loading capacity of a person with flat back would be 60 percent less than that of a person maintaining a proper lumbar lordosis, before causing damage to her/his spinal disc, assuming all else being equal.

Using a person with flat back as a reference, her weight lifting capacity would increase by 150 percent, if she's able to adopt a proper lumbar curvature. This phenomena is further exaggerated in the case of people with advanced degeneration in the spinal discs, (good curvature) it will help improve the spine's loading capacity by far more than 150 percent because the spinal discs are far less capable of properly distributing the spinal pressure across the surface of the spinal disc. See the illustration of pressure distribution in the above image.

Simply put: A healthy lumbar lordosis (curvature of lower back) will make your spine 150 percent stronger. Speaking from a spinal biomechanical perspective, this is true for anybody, in most upright positions, especially when weight lifting or obesity is involved.

What is a good spinal curvature? To most people, it is your natural curvature in your lower back before back pain or injury, when standing on level ground. Your eyes comfortably looking straight, forward to the horizon. And with no shoes on your feet.

You may find this definition a mouthful, or even lacking precision. The fact is that a good lower back curvature is different from individual to individual. A person with a flat back growing up healthy may be plagued with back pain if a curve is forced on him. A person with a scoliosis (abnormal lateral curvature of the spine) growing up, but otherwise healthy, may suffer from severe back pain if a medical procedure is applied on her back to straighten the whole spine. So a natural posture or curvature is very individualistic.

Many activities may cause the healthy curvature in your back to be compromised, such as:
- Driving a vehicle,
- Piloting an airplane,
- Working in an office environment,
- Taking care of a patient as a nurse,
- Treating patients as a dentist or a dental hygienist,
- Handling packages,

- Laying carpeting,
- Doing a machining job,
- Doing a construction job,
- Planting flowers,
- Enjoying a ball game in a stadium, or
- Watching a TV program while sitting on a couch.

The list goes on and on. Most of our daily activities that require sitting or bending our back forward compromises the healthy curvature and wellbeing of our lower back to some degree.

If you sit for a prolonged period, consider using a proper back support. The ideal back support must offer all following three key ingredients:

- Customizability: our bodies are not built equal. Our back has different shapes. Most importantly the curvatures of our body differ from one to the next. The perfect back support for one person may be terrible to another person.

  Furthermore, our seats are different. The back of a car seat is radically different from that of a couch. A perfect back support for your car seat will make you feel miserable on a sofa.

  Your back support must be easily customizable to suit your back and your seat.

- Dynamic support: our body is not built for still sitting. Your back support must be able to accommodate and encourage the movement of your back. Deprived of motion over a period of time, even the most ergonomic glove will make your hand feel terrible. The same shall happen to your back.

  In general, back support made of static substances such as foam (including memory foam), fibres, plastics or wood are incapable of accommodate or facilitate movement in the back. The most practical and successful substance used to offer dynamic support is air. Theoretically, water or gel should also offer you dynamic support. However they are too difficult and cumbersome to use in daily life.

Air based back support shall be the focus of your search for an idea support for your back.

- Strong support: only strong support can help prevent slouching, and maintain a good spinal alignment. Any device that loses its support against the pressure of the back is not strong enough and is not able to help maintain a health spinal alignment. Foam (including memory foam) or fibre based back support tend to compress and lose their support behind the back, and are not suable to support your back.

You may consider the JazzRX dynamic orthopedic back support or Qi Orthopedic Pillow for this purpose, because they offer all three above mentioned key qualities of an idea back support.

If your work or daily life requires you to frequently bend your back forward, you need to frequently interrupt your back bending activity, ideally once every 20-minutes. If you can't have such frequent breaks of back bending activity, you need to consider assistive devices that help you to at least reduce the tension and stress in your back while bending your back.

3. Use Your Muscles not Your Spine. Don't Slouch.

Muscles are to be strengthened, not to be weakened. However, often the reverse happens with most of the people who are susceptible to back pain. And when that happens, the load will be concentrated on the spine. The spine is forced to take on more. Its biomechanics worsen, and its wear and tear increases.

Slouching is a typical action we do, that weakens the back muscles. When you slouch, your abdominal muscles are compressed and your back muscles and ligaments are slowly stretched. With prolonged slouching, your back muscles, especially the deep stabilizing muscles, and ligaments will be out of tone and will be loosened and weakened. The loosening of stabilizing muscles and ligaments eventually contributes to damage or injury of the spinal discs.

On the other hand, your slouching also worsens the pressure distribution of your spinal discs and causes peak pressure on your spinal discs to emerge, especially in the lower back. Such peak pressure significantly surpasses the corresponding pressure when you are not slouching, to increase the wear and tear of your spine. Over time such increased wear and tear of your spine will also lead to damage or injury of your spine, especially your spinal discs in your lower back.

Furthermore, slouch begets and worsens the slouch itself. Slouching is a self-reinforcing and continuously worsening process, just like the tilting of the Pisa Tower is a self-reinforcing and continuously worsening process.

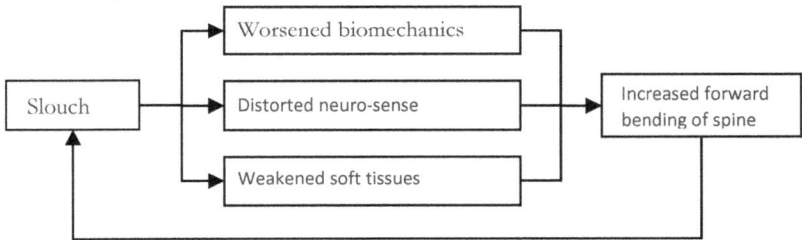

Source: Patrick Lee

Fig. 3.2

4. Use Your Legs and Breath, not Your Back

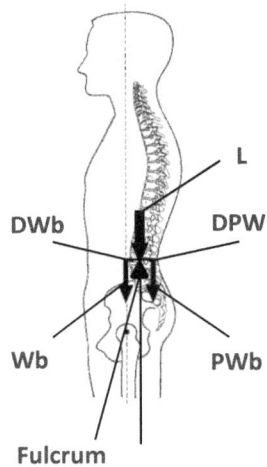

When lifting heavy objects, keep your back straight and hold a full breath, instead of hunching your back and holding a soft or no breath. And use your legs to push up your body lifting with your legs, instead of extending your spine upwards to lift with your back.

When you pick up a newspaper off the ground, you want to bend your knees and lower your body to reach for it, instead of bending your back to reach for it.

For an adult with 160 LB body weight, the simple act of bending your back forward to reach the floor with your

Source: Patrick Lee

Fig. 3.3

163

hand and reverse your upper body up will increase the load in your back muscles from 80 LB to 1,120 LB, because the DWb had been increased 14 folds. This increases the load on your spinal discs from 160 LB close to 1,200 LB – 7.5 folds increase, although you may not notice this incredible increase in your spinal load.

In the case of a male adult with an average body height of 5 foot and 10 inches, for each pound of weight you pick or lift up by first leaning your back forward and bending your spine back up, instead of your legs, and without holding a strong breath, the load in your lower back muscles increases by a increment of 22 LB because in such case DWe is typically increased to 22 times DPW. This means that our body has a factor of 22 in enlarging the weight we pick up when

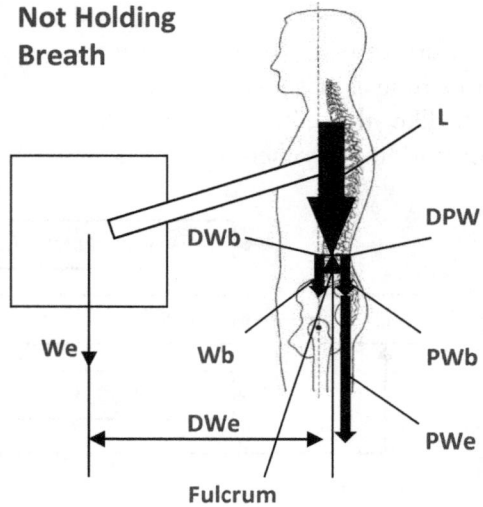

Source: Patrick Lee

Fig. 3.4

using our spine without holding a strong breath. However this amplifying factor can be dramatically reduced.

If you keep heavy object close to your body but not holding a full breath, the above mentioned amplifying factor can still be as high as 15 – meaning for each pound of weight you hold in your hands, the stress in your back muscles shall increase by 15 LB.

Holding a strong breath when lifting heavy weight can greatly reduce the stress in your back and spine. First, it completely changes the system of Moment Equilibrium in your body by shifting the pivot or fulcrum forward to the abdomen muscles from the centre of the spinal discs, and dramatically reduce the muscle tension required to balance the external weight, hence the load on your spinal discs. Second, it create an additional load bearing structure (air chamber) to share the load with your spine, heance further reduce the load on your spinal discs.

- Wb – the weight of your body above the level of the vertebra or disc measured

- We – the external weigh you lift or carry

- PWb – phantom weight your spine takes due to your own body biomechanics and posture

- PWe – phantom weight your spine takes due to the way you lift or carry external weight.

- DWb – the distance between the centre of the abdomen muscles and the gravity center line of the upper body.

- DWe – the horizontal distance between the centre of the abdomen muscles and the centre of your load-bearing hand which shall roughly be aligned with the gravity center line of the weight you lift.

- DPW – the distance between the centre of the abdomen muscles and the stabilizing muscles.

$PWb = 0$ (because Wb is at the same side of fulcrum as back muscles)

$$L \text{ (spine)} + L \text{ (air chamber)} = (Wb + PWb) + (We + PWe)$$

$$We \times DWe = Wb \times DWb + PWe \times DPW$$

$$PWe = (We \times DWe - Wb \times DWb)/DPW$$

Compared with not holding a strong breath while lifting weight, when an average adult holds a strong breath while lifting weight, he would increase the leverage of his back muscle by 9 folds, while reducing the leverage of the external weight by 30%. Simultaneously he also turns the body weight into a friendly force in counter balancing the external weight while increasing its leverage by 7 folds.

If you keep heavy object close to your body and hold a full breath, you shall reduce the amplifying factor as discusses before by a stunning 93 percent – down from 15 (not holding a strong breath) to 1 or less (holding a strong breath). This means, by holding a strong breath, each pound of weight you hold in your hands would only cause one pound or less increase in the stress in your back muscles, instead of 15 pounds.

Holding your breath also creates a weight bearing air chamber inside your body to share the load that otherwise would be purely loaded on your spinal discs. This is particularly important in such cases as weight lifting competition. It is, however, important to point out that people need to maintain a health lower back curvature for the internal air chamber to function the best, because the internal air chamber has a tendency to destabilizing the spine in the case of flat backs or reversed lower back curvature.

It is important to realize that if you simply keep heavy objects close to your body, but do not hold a breath or only hold an empty breath, the amplifying factor would only marginally reduce from 22 (by keeping weight forward of the body with arms fully stretched) to 15 (by keeping heavy object touching the body). Keeping a heavy object close to your body is only one part of the story.

As you can see from the above analysis, it is important to remember to not only keep heavy objects as close to your body as you can, but also to keep a healthy curvature in your back, while holding a strong full breath, before pushing up with your legs to lift the heavy object. If you are an amateur or professional weight lifter, a heavy material handler, or a fitness enthusiast, your must remind yourself on all three points, instead of the conventional wisdom of the single point of holding the weight close to your body only.

5. Minimize Forward Head Posture and Hyperkyphosis

Unfortunately, most activities we do at work or at home require our head to be leaning forward. From working on a computer, to reading a book, to writing a text on a smart phone, to talking to someone shorter than you, to having breakfast, to playing video games, planting a flower, cooking a meal, or even brushing your teeth. If you are not careful, the cumulative effect of these activities will easily create a persistent medical condition called Forward Head Posture (a.k.a. Anterior Head Carriage, or Anterior Head Translation).

With such a condition, your brain considers the forward head posture as a perfectly normal and correct posture. Your brain will not only accept such posture as a good one for you, but also directs your body into such a posture, even when you do not have a need for such a posture, to reinforce the permanence of this pain-causing medical condition.

Forward head posture is a habitual problem. It develops unknowingly over a prolonged period. When you become aware of it, it is likely to have crept on you for too long. It may make you look less attractive. It may cause nagging pain and discomfort in your neck and your upper back. It may cause severe headache. It may distract your focus and attention. It may significantly reduce your vital capacity. It may cause premature aging and spinal degeneration. It may lead you to hunch your back, as forward head posture not only begets forward head posture, it also causes and begets hunched back (hyperkyphosis). It may lead to your struggle and frustration in treating the pain. It may lead to your suffering from the side effects of drugs you take to combat the pain. It may lead to depression, and other ailments.

Forward head posture may start as a benign process, yet it certainly has serious, even devastating consequences.

You can easily check to see whether you have forward head posture. Try the following three-second test now:

1. Simply stand with your back against a straight wall, with no protrusion from the top to the lower end.
2. Make sure your buttocks are in touch with the wall.
3. Gently pull both of your feet to touch the wall with your heels while making sure that your legs are straight.
4. Gently open up your shoulders and touch the wall with the full length of your shoulder.
5. Finally, gently reverse your head to touch the wall with the back of your head, while keeping your chin in, so your face is towards your front horizontally, instead of up into the sky.

How do you feel now? Are you able to do it easily or without any struggle?

People with minor or no forward head posture or a hunched back should be able to do this simple test easily, quickly, and comfortably.

If you experience any difficulty in doing this test, especially with your shoulder and head touching the wall, chances are that your forward head posture or hunched back or both may already be in an advanced stage.

It is important to realize that forward head posture and hunched back conditions are not exclusive to adults. With the prevalence of iPads, iPhones, and other mobile devices, such serious conditions are increasingly present among teenagers.

Check your neck posture today. Ask your loved ones and your children to do the same, today. Take actions to minimize and prevent it starting today. One ounce of prevention is better than a pound of cure down the road. Nip the problem in the bud, before it becomes too advanced.

6. Keep an Open Chest

A closed chest worsens the biomechanics of your neck. With a closed chest, your head will be forced to tilt forward as soon as you are not consciously aware of it. A closed chest or forward rolling shoulders often lead to forward head posture and the associated neck pain and upper back pain.

When your shoulders roll forward and your chest is closed, your head will tend to shift forward no matter what exercise or therapy you do to help your neck.

A healthy and open chest is the prerequisite for a healthy neck.

7. Maintain Your Core and Postural Stability.

Your core stability is the foundation of your postural stability. A poor postural stability is a sure recipe for poor posture, poor body biomechanics, abnormal muscle and ligament tensions, and stretches, worsened stress in your spine, increased wear and tear to your spine, premature spinal degeneration, unnecessary spinal injury, and eventually back pain, sooner or later.

Exercise your core regularly. There are many exercises that are effective in helping you develop, maintain or enhance your core stability.

You can participate in physical therapy exercises that often use stability balls, or participate in Pilates lessons, or Yoga, or Tai Chi practices.

2

8 Right Lifestyles You Must Adopt

Lifestyle plays an indisputably critical role on the quality of modern human life. In a 2012 report, Dr. Doug Manuel, Senior Scientist, Clinical Epidemiology, Ottawa Hospital Research Institute, pointed out that six out of 10 deaths in Ontario, Canada, are linked to five controllable habits: smoking, alcohol consumption, physical inactivity, unhealthy eating, and stress. By eliminating these risk factors, you can add seven more years to your life, while adding even more life to your years.

In 2014, Dr. Doug Manuel published a follow up report stating that severe issues associated with four out of the five habits, (smoking, alcohol dependency, physical inactivity, and an unhealthy diet) could advance a person's initial hospitalization by 25-years for men with exposure to all four risk factors, beginning hospitalization at age of 35 instead of 60 for men with no health risks, and 20-years for women beginning at age of 38 instead of 58 for women with no health risks. In other words, issues with these habits could rob a quarter to a third of your quality of life from you.

Want to know what your life expectancy could be with your current lifestyle? Get a free assessment at www.projectbiglife.ca

which was developed with extensive analysis of 70,000 individuals and 900,000 in-hospital days. (Note: this author is not affiliated with this website, nor with Dr. Manual, nor with the Ottawa Hospital Research Institute.)

All five of these controllable habits have also been linked to back pain. Effective mitigation of smoking, alcohol consumption, physical inactivity, unhealthy eating, and stress will effectively help you enhance your spinal health, relieve and prevent back pain.

1.   Maintain a Healthy Body Weight

Eat healthy, keep body weight in a healthy range. Avoid obesity.

In the case of a body with obesity, not only the body weight that a disc in the lower back has to support increases, but also the center of gravity of the upper body shifts further forward, away from the spine, which dramatically increases the stress in the muscles in your lower back that are responsible to hold your back upright.

If, for example, the corresponding body weight increases from 80 LB to 120 LB, and the distance between the gravity line and the center of the disc increases 20 percent, the counter balancing muscle force will have to increase to 144 LB. The resulting total load of the disc suddenly jumps to 264 LB. A whole 104 LB or 65 percent more spinal load for just 40 LB more weight in the upper body. Along with the dramatically increased load on the spine, the supporting condition of the spine significantly worsens.

The spine has to tilt further backward like a tilted building. Imagine an office tower. Now, what would happen to the structure of the office tower when an additional block the size of more than half of the original office tower is dropped on top, while at the same time the office tower is placed tilted on the ground? Imagine how much this office tower has to struggle not to fall down. Imagine how much fear you would have going into such a tower to work. And imagine now that office tower is this body with obesity of only 40 LB more than normal.

As we all know obesity often creates far more than 40 LB in the upper body. If the above described picture is terrifying enough, imagine what would happen to the body if it creates 60 LB, even 80 LB more weight to the upper body (very common obesity conditions).

Is it of any surprise to know that people with obesity are often afflicted by back aches and pains?

Unfortunately, obesity is not a static process. Obesity begets obesity! It's a vicious circle that is hard to break.

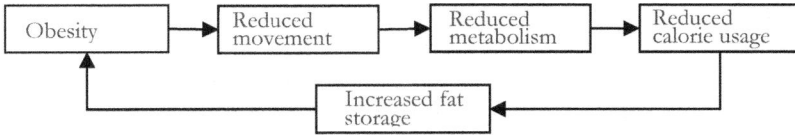

source: Patrick Lee

Fig. 3.6

Obesity also often leads to a reduced level of physical activity and exercises, which reduces body metabolism and calorie consumption, which in turn increases storage of fat in the body and further increases the body.

There are also social factors at play. Obese people tend to socialize more with other obese people, while reducing contact with people without obesity. That is why you often see a whole family of people who are obese. You may say that it is because of the special gene of the family. Such logic may lead to some explanations about the obesity in the children. But how could you explain the obesity in a husband or wife?

You may say: "Obesity is a medical condition. I don't want to be obese. And I have done everything possible to get rid of it. But I simply put on weight even if I just drink water."

Let's face it, obesity is only a medical condition because the medical community and the big pharmaceutical companies have medicalized the condition this way. Simply by looking around your home, you will find that the medicalization is wrong and its rational is against the laws of nature. There can be no accumulation of energy without energy input.

What would happen to a pot of beautiful flowers if you don't water it for a month? It will dry up. Has anyone ever seen a flower or a tree to grow into a gigantic size without sufficient water supply? Has anyone ever seen a long-starved child or mother being overweight? Even a cactus in the desert needs a regular water supply to grow. Even camels need food to survive their long journeys.

A living organism can't grow without input of energy. If this is such a primitive truth that even children know it, then why do we, grownups, consider that our body weight would grow even without input of energy? Stop fooling yourself, even though the medical community or big pharma may want you to do so. I am not saying that you need to starve yourself to address obesity. There are more elegant, comfortable, and cost effective ways for that. See below.

Surgery has been considered the most effective solution to obesity. In the province of British Columbia, Canada, where all such operations are paid for by the provincial government, the waiting list is extremely long and the waiting time for a weight loss operation is up to 10-years. Why does everyone want an operation? Because they were told that operations are effective. But have they thought about the fact that the weight would return after operation, if their way of life is unchanged? Operations are effective to reduce weight in the short-term; but not effective to resolve obesity for the longer-term, because it only addresses the symptom instead of the cause.

In an era when we are all made to think that anything clinically proven is good, anything not clinically proven is not good, we must realize that clinically proven is not always good. Operations for obesity are one of the best examples. Thoughtless prescriptions and applications of pain killers is another.

In life, many good things can't currently be proven, as with the approach based on chemicals and metals. To address the cause is always more challenging than addressing the symptoms. To address the causes in a safe and organic way is even more challenging. What would you opt for, an approach that has been proven universally to merely treat symptoms or an approach that has been individually proven to treat the root cause?

The #MadBack NDANC (No Diet and No Cost) Regimen for Weight Loss:

1. Drink a LARGE glass of plain water 30-minutes, before any meal.*
2. Have an ALL vegetable salad with low calorie dressing, ahead of each main course.*
3. Cut out ALL high calorie gravies and sauces.*
4. Chew a MINIMUM of 20-times with each bite.*
5. Eat until 70 to 80 percent full ONLY.*

6.   Use low sodium (salt) in food and food preparation.*
7.   Do NOT have dinner at least two hours before bed time.*
8.   Eat NO more than three meals a day.*
9.   Eat NO desert.*
10. Eat NO snacks NOR sweets.*
11. Eat NO junk food NOR transfat.*
12. Drink NO sugared NOR sweetened drinks, soda, juice, tea or coffee.*
13. If you feel very hungry before a meal time, do something that demands concentration.
14. Go for a 20-minute walk after EACH meal.
15. Go to bed NO later than 10 pm.
16. Listen to music from a PURE audio player for at least three-hours a day.
17. Watch TV NO more than one-hour a day.
18. Get up and move more whenever you can, the more and the more intense, the better.
19. STOP ANY other weight loss regiment while following this plan.*
20. DOUBLE and then RE-DOUBLE your socialization with people with NO obesity.
21. Do NOT stop following this plan within six-months.
22. REJECT the notion that obesity is a medical condition.*

* *highest priority To-Dos.*

Source: developed by Patrick Lee

Fig. 3.7

By simply following points #1 through point #5 of the above regimen for six-months, this author easily lost 30 LB of body weight. Imagine how much weight you could lose by following the complete regimen stated above.

Best of all, this regimen needs no diet, costs no money, involves no chemicals, and requires no surgery. It is all natural and only requires a little will power, knowledge, patience, and discipline, at a level any adult is capable of. Where there is a will, there is a way. Besides, compared with the suffering and pain associated with obesity, the little patience and discipline required are truly insignificant.

"But this is too good to be true because I have tried many expensive diets and I still have the weight problem." And a recent study indicates that only 5 percent of obese people have succeeded in losing some weight. Some doctors even give up on the idea of helping patients lose weight and believe that weight, once gained, can't be lost, and even term it as an "unfortunate truth," while realizing that weight gain is mostly a habitual issue.

The truth is simple. Without addressing the root cause, weight loss is indeed hard and hardly sustainable. Commercial diets are designed to make profit. They have to be expensive, otherwise they are not able to make money. They have to ask you to consume certain things they supply, otherwise no money could be made. They have to ask you to follow some strange routines otherwise they will not be able to stand out to catch your interest. Despite all of these commercial considerations, if they do not address fundamental mechanisms of obesity, they can't help you.

What is the fundamental mechanism of obesity, you ask? Simple. It is about how you help your body control its cravings. People with obesity may have a slower metabolism. It is true that, according to a 2013 study by the Welcome Trust-MRC Institute of Metabolic Science in Cambridge, and Cambridge University, UK, mutations in the KSR2 gene (also known as "the fat gene") could reduce the ability of cells to metabolize glucose and fatty acids, which provides energy, and leads to higher appetite and lower metabolism.

"Up until now, the genes we have identified that control body weight have largely affected appetite," said Professor Sadaf Farooqi, University of Cambridge. "This gene also increases appetite but it also causes a slow metabolic rate."

But such gene mutation is only present in two percent of the severely obese population. Most people with obesity have no problem with either metabolism or gene mutation. Controlling appetite remains the central challenge in the fight against obesity.

If you want to control your body weight with the help of any drug, diet or surgery, you must ask yourself if you can continue to take the drug or eat the special diet, or repeat that surgery, for the rest of your life. If the answer is no, you need to seriously consider alternatives to drugs, diets, and surgeries.

The NDNC regimen above is specially designed to help you easily, quickly, comfortably, and affordably control your appetite. It makes nobody any money, except you – the reader of this book and effective loser of weight.

To benefit from the plan, you don't have to do all the points on day one. A gradual approach would be better for your system.

Begin with, "drinking one big glass of water 30-minutes prior to each meal." Add only one further point each day. Make a ritual out of your new routine. Rituals dramatically increase the implementation, the quality, and the power of the routines. The more ritualistic, the more sacred and the more efficient and effective your routine becomes. Most great masters, fighters and athletes follow some of their routines ritualistically.

The following is a progressive check list to assure your gradual and complete implementation of the effective plan.

	1	2	3	4	5	6	7	8	9	10	11	12	13	14	15	16	17	18	19	20	21	22
1	x	X	x	x	x	x	x	x	x	x	x	x	x	x	x	x	x	x	x	x	x	x
2		X	x	x	x	x	x	x	x	x	x	x	x	x	x	x	x	x	x	x	x	x
3			x	x	x	x	x	x	x	x	x	x	x	x	x	x	x	x	x	x	x	x
4				x	x	x	x	x	x	x	x	x	x	x	x	x	x	x	x	x	x	x
5					x	x	x	x	x	x	x	x	x	x	x	x	x	x	x	x	x	x
6						x	x	x	x	x	x	x	x	x	x	x	x	x	x	x	x	x
7							x	x	x	x	x	x	x	x	x	x	x	x	x	x	x	x
8								x	x	x	x	x	x	x	x	x	x	x	x	x	x	x
9									x	x	x	x	x	x	x	x	x	x	x	x	x	x
10										x	x	x	x	x	x	x	x	x	x	x	x	x
11											x	x	x	x	x	x	x	x	x	x	x	x
12												x	x	x	x	x	x	x	x	x	x	x
13													x	x	x	x	x	x	x	x	x	x
14														x	x	x	x	x	x	x	x	x
15															x	x	x	x	x	x	x	x
16																x	x	x	x	x	x	x
17	x	X	x	x	x	x	x	x	x	x	x	x	x	x	x	x	x	x	x	x	x	x
18																		x	x	x	x	x
19	x	X	x	x	x	x	x	x	x	x	x	x	x	x	x	x	x	x	x	x	x	x
20	x	X	x	x	x	x	x	x	x	x	x	x	x	x	x	x	x	x	x	x	x	x

Source: Patrick Lee

Fig. 3.8

You may say, "I am not obese. This phenomena does not apply to me."

Well, do you work in an office? Do you sit? If you do, the same phenomena also applies to you. And the chances are you do sit, as we all do. You sit to work on a computer, you sit to have your meals, you sit to watch your ball games, you sit to enjoy your favorite Netflix programs.

So how would that terrible phenomena apply to you? Here is the how and why.

The gravity of your upper body moves forward when you sit down – often as much as three times as much as when you stand. The back muscles have to exert three times the force to counter balance the same weight in the upper body. If, as discussed above, the muscle force was 80 LB when standing up, the same muscle force is now increased to 240 LB. And the total load on your spinal discs has increased from 160 LB to 320 LB – even more than those in the cases of obesity.

Is it any surprise to know that according to the Workplace Safety and Insurance Board (WSIB) in Ontario, Canada, sitting is a leading cause of back pain, second only to heavy weight lifting?

Of course, in the above case of a person with obesity sitting down, and they do tend to sit more than normal people due to the obesity, the total disc pressure increases close to 500 LB from 264 LB.

As a result, from the total spinal load perspective, sitting affects the spine more negatively than obesity. This is not to say that you should choose obesity over sitting, partly because sitting is inevitable.

From the same token, one could also understand that sitting is only for the legs, not for the back. Simply sitting down is not the solution for you if you have problems with your back and you want to have a break to relieve it.

2. Lower Heels and Right Fashions

Pride knows no pain. However, if you are health conscious and want your beauty to be sustainable, you want to pay attention to the right fashion.

Clothes need to be comfortable. Tight clothes may restrict your blood flow and affect your body mechanics and posture negatively.

Also, be reminded, that there is no reason for shoes to have heels at all, except to make one appear taller, or to make the shoes wear a bit longer. Health wise, heels are bad, bad, bad!!! The higher the heels, the worse it is to your health, and your back. Actually, in most situations, high heels only make one look less beautiful and attractive, especially viewed sideways.

"Oh, we know high heels are bad. But …" argued my on air hosts, one day when I was on QVC, an American television shopping channel.

Okay, I give in because I understand that sometimes ladies just need to opt for high heels. But please also do what my on air hosts do – take the high heels off shortly after their on air presentation. It is nice and cute to see them walking around in the studio in their bare feet.

You can prepare a pair of low or no heel shoes as alternatives to your high heels. Wear them on your way to and from your office. Wear them when you are not in the public's view. Keep a pair of light portable no heel shoes for travel or in your office or cubicle. Minimize the time in which you wear your high heels, as much as possible.

3. Get Thy Stress Under Control

According to the American National Institute of Health and the American Institute of Science, Technology and Public Policy, 90 percent of illness is caused or complicated by stress. Stress has reached an epidemic level and scale in America. Most people perceive the intensity of their own stress at level 7 to 8 on a 1 to 10 point scale, with 10 representing "completely stressed out." Stress has become a strong contributor to both high medical costs and poor medical outcomes.

Stress has long been linked to back pain. Our back is like a thermometer to our physical, mental, and emotional stress. In many cases, the brain is the origin of pain in your back, which has been repeatedly proven in clinical studies.

According to the American Psychological Association, there are three main types of stresses:

- *Acute stresses* are short term stresses and the most common form of stress. It is driven by the demand and pressure from recent past events or near future events. Small and infrequent doses, such as a few per day, of acute stress may be a good thing that may make your life more exciting and help you achieve more. Too many or too much acute stresses may generate negative effects.

Acute stresses may involve emotional stress, such as anger or irritability, anxiety, and depression. Such stresses may have physical manifestations, such as tension headache, back pain, jaw pain, and tensed muscles that increase the risk of pulled muscles, tendons, and ligaments. Such stresses may also affect the function of your stomach, gut and bowel, creating heartburn, diarrhea, irritable bowel, and so on. They can also lead to cardiovascular problems, such as high blood pressure, dizziness, migraine headache, chest pain.

There is no such thing as a stress free life. However, enough is enough. Keep a healthy limit on the frequency and intensity of your acute stresses, and actively use them to your advantage.

- *Episodic acute stress* emerges when acute stresses become too frequent. If acute stresses are more caused by external factors, episodic acute stresses are more caused by the internal factors of its sufferers. Some people are so ambitious that they take on too much and everything is at the risk of falling off of their plates. Others may be so disorganized that they are always rushing, yet always late for something. These people tend to be short-tempered, irritable, anxious, tense, and hostile, which often spills over to people surrounding them, to create a vicious emotional circle. The workplace or even family may become stressful places to them and those around them.

Episodic acute stress also comes from continued and endless worries. Sufferers of such stress tend to worry about everything on a continued basis. They tend to be more anxious and depressed. If such a person is afflicted by back pain, a perfect storm of viscous pain-worry-depression-pain circle may take place. Because the lifestyle and personality of these sufferers are so ingrained, they often don't see anything wrong with their situation.

Keep things in perspective. Open your mind to constructive suggestions. Don't stress yourself too much. Your health and life will not get better because of the stresses that you create for yourself.

- *Chronic stress* emerges when stress becomes constant over a prolonged period. It is the worst form of stress and tends to be entirely negative and detrimental to your mind and body. Chronic pain, chronic diseases, fear or anxiety from childhood, poor relationships, and financial constrains can all be sources of chronic stress.

Chronic stress wears your mind and body down. It weakens your heart and immune system. It increases the inflammation inside your body. It limits your creative thinking, your achievement, your joy, your happiness, your sexuality, your expression of love, your heart, your back and more. Ninety percent of today's diseases are caused or complicated by stress, mostly by chronic stress. Chronic stress to your body and mind is like little drops of water that, in the short-term, seem harmless. However, over the long-term, they can drill a hole in through hard rock.

Due to its chronic nature, chronic stresses often become invisible to their sufferers. Sufferers don't even realize the existence of such stress. If you have chronic back pain of unknown cause, you may wish to examine and assess your state of stress. If identified, you can apply simple, natural, and low cost ways, such as transcendental meditation, yoga or engagement with supportive friends, to combat it.

Stress is not an entirely subjective matter. Its physical manifestation and responses can be objectively measured by the relatively new Heart Rate Variability (HRV) technology. Instead of measuring the number of heart beats per minute, HRV technology measures variation of the time interval between your heartbeats. The clinical relevance of HRV was first reported in 1965, by Hon and Lee, on their finding that fetal distress was preceded by alterations in time intervals between heartbeats before any noticeable change occurred in the heart rate itself.

Research indicates that higher HRV value is linked to better health and a higher level of fitness, while lower HRV is linked to stress, fatigue, poor health or fitness. HRV technology puts your heart under a magnifier for closer analysis and monitoring, and reveals insight about your health that is not obtainable from simple heart rate monitors. According to the Journal of American College of Cardiology, measurement of heart rate variability (HRV) has become an important research tool for both clinical and basic scientists.

HRV technology has found its way into a large number of clinics and become available for access by the general public. If you are not sure about your level of stress, especially if you suffer from chronic stress, you may wish to visit a doctor to take a HRV test.

Manage your mental and emotional stress from work, home, and relationships. Do not drive yourself too hard mentally. Don't load yourself too much emotionally. Don't push yourself too hard work wise.

Distance yourself from environments filled with negative emotions. Look at the fuller half of the glass. Look at the brighter side of your life. Don't sweat about small things. Don't be too ambitious. Don't stretch your limit too much. Stay away from people with negative or egotistic personalities. Your back pain is your body's way of saying, "things are not right and get me out of the stress." Stop being too perfect. Aiming for perfection in life is a paradox, because it inevitably leads to imperfections in major parts of your life. Life is about compromise. A perfectly imperfect life is a more beneficial goal for you, at least for the health of your back.

If you can't eliminate your source of stress, at least you can reduce your level of stress. Meditation is a great way to de-stress yourself. In a randomized clinical study, published in Hypertension by R.H. Schneider and others, stress-reducing transcendental meditation was 2.5 times more effective in reducing systolic and diastolic blood pressure than conventional relaxation. The effects of transcendental meditation were comparable to standard pharmacological treatment, but without the adverse side-effects or high costs of hypertensive drugs.

According to an article published in Psychosomatic Medicine, by D.W. Orme-Johnson and others, the statistics of the health insurance company Blue Cross/Blue Shield showed an average 50 percent reduction in medical utilization across all 16 disease categories in people practicing the Transcendental Meditation program compared to people who didn't.

Walking, exercising, good sleep, being in nature, listening to happy music, attending comedy shows, and enjoying a belly laugh can also help balance your brain. Mind and body is a whole entity. Positive bodily sensations and relaxation can help the brain to respond positively and relax.

4. Smoke Not

Smoking is not only bad for your lungs. Numerous studies have shown cigarette smoking is closely associated with back pain and disc diseases. Smoking is a leading cause for spinal degeneration. Researchers found that both reduction in the density of vascular buds and narrowing of the vascular lumen (artery) caused by nicotine results in decreased oxygen tension, leading to decreased synthesis of proteoglycan and collagen, thus facilitating degeneration of the disc.

In a 53-year period study that started in 1949, 1,337 of doctors that graduated from John Hopkins medical school in the period of 1948 to 1964, were analyzed regarding the development of chronic lower back pain, lumbar herniated nucleus propolsus, and lumbar spondylosis, among them, in relation to their lifestyles. The result was published in 2001.

Dr. Nicholas U. Ahn, associate professor of orthopaedic surgery at Case Western Reserve University School of Medicine, and his co-authors of this study found that chronic lower back pain was clearly linked to both smoking and hypertension, with hypertension having doubled the effect, and that lumbar spondylosis was linked with smoking, hypertension, obesity, and other atherosclerosis risk factors that cause hardening and inflammation in blood vessel walls. This study concluded that chronic hardening and inflammation of segmental arteries is a cause of lumbar spine disease, lower back pain, and lumbar spine degeneration. Smoking is a significant cause to the hardening and inflammation of arteries, hence spinal degeneration and back pain.

5. Eat Healthy

You may have heard of the phrase: "you are what you eat." Indeed it has a lot of truth in itself because, after all, eating is like breathing and sleeping, the most fundamental functions in human survival.

To eat healthy, you need to pay attention to both what you eat and how you eat. Most people know to avoid junk foods. But there is more to that. And as they say: "it is not what you say, it is how you say it," that counts in effective communication. By the same token, "it is not what you eat, it is how you eat it," that counts for your health.

What you eat:

- Avoid junk food, trans-fat rich food.

- Eat anti-inflammatory foods. (See more details in section "The Right Nutrition" below.)

How you eat:
- Regular schedule.
- Quality breakfast.
- No late dinner.
- Chew properly.
- Moderate amounts.
- Right combinations.

6. Reduce Alcohol Consumption

Alcohol consumption could also contribute to back pain. By pooling and analyzing data from 26 clinical studies, a team of researchers found that alcohol dependency was linked to complex and chronic back pain by studies in a report published in 2013.

While moderate alcohol consumption may be beneficial to your health, alcohol dependency may not. If you have, to some degree, developed a dependency on alcohol consumption, seek help immediately. Getting help for problems with alcohol can have important effects on your life, not only on your back pain.

3

12 Critical Body Care Approaches You Must Take

An ounce of care is better than a pound of treatment. One of the key reasons why back pain is troubling almost one in every person is that the back and spine are mostly taken for granted. We as a society give dramatically less attention to the back and spinal health than to the teeth, while back and spinal health is far more important than that of our teeth. Back problems are far more difficult and costly to treat than those of teeth.

The fact is that, if you don't invest in your own health today, you will be investing in doctors and pharmaceutical companies tomorrow. The good news is that the investments in yourself today doesn't have to be monetary. It can be a little effort, a little more awareness, a little more knowledge, a little will to do better, a little prevention, and a little regular care.

In contrast, the investments in doctors and pharmaceutical companies tomorrow will most likely be a more costly, prolonged suffering, persistent agony, withdrawal from your favorite activities, even an interruption of your career and loss of income.

Which investment would you prefer? The investments in yourself today, or the investments in doctors and pharmaceutical companies tomorrow?

To avoid your spine under living you, you must take proper care, now.

1. Sit Right

In today's sedentary society whose people spend 80 to 90 percent of their daily awakening time sitting in seats, chairs, cars or airplanes. Sitting is, according to the Workers Safety and Insurance Board of Ontario, Canada (WSIB), the leading cause for back pain second only to heavy weight lifting. Sitting right is critical to your back and spinal health.

Generally speaking, there are two main issues with incorrect sitting. The first issue is slouching, which destroys the proper spinal alignment and impedes blood flow, and increases wear and tear of the spine. The second issue is physical inactivity in your trunk and pelvis, which causes the deep stabilizing muscles in the back to tense and often leads to stiffness, pain or fatigue in the back. The physical inactivity has also been linked to many other health problems, such as obesity, diabetes, cardiovascular problems, breast cancers, colon cancers, and premature death.

The physical activity of your trunk and pelvis is of utmost importance to the proper functioning of your inner organs, your metabolism, your hormones and your immune system, and the general biochemical and biomechanical balancing processes of your body in which your body's physiological system maintains its internal stability, based on the coordinated response of its parts to any situation or stimulus that would tend to disturb its normal condition or function – a process formally called Human Homeostasis. This is main reason that many devastating diseases such as obesity, cardiovascular diseases, colon cancer, breast cancer and premature death have been attributed to prolonged sitting.

Simply kicking your legs or moving your arms without involving your trunk while sitting is insufficient. You may say: "how, then, would taking a break to walk help me? I use my legs and not my trunk while walking." The reality is that your trunk and pelvis are actively involved while walking. As you take each step, your body weight shifts from one leg to the other. Your pelvis moves to accommodate this shifting process. Since your pelvis is the foundation of your trunk, your trunk also moves to accommodate the movement of your pelvis. That is why walking is so helpful to your health.

It is critical to reduce both slouching and physical inactivity while sitting.

Try to sit upright, avoid slouching, and maintain the gravity centers of your head and trunk in the same vertical line wherever possible. Unfortunately, most chairs and sofas are not built to support a good posture. Car seats, air plane seats, and the expensive big executive chairs are often the typical examples of poor ergonomic design for posture.

Properly designed posture aids can be highly beneficial. You may want to look into good back supports and postural seats.

You also need to use your body correctly. For example, if you need to lean your body forward to reach something deep on your desk, shift your body forward from your hip, instead of bending your back.

The other important aspect of right sitting is to reduce physical inactivity. Try to take frequent breaks from sitting whenever you can. You can set a reminder on your smart phone. Some people even use their bladder to remind them, by bringing a big bottle of water to their desk and drinking from it frequently. In time your bladder will be full and remind, or even force you, to get up for a break.

Good dynamic seating can help you break down your physical inactivity effectively, because it can continuously stimulate your body to move, subconsciously. In a sense, such dynamic seating will eliminate physical inactivity in your trunk.

From the above discussion, you realize that traditional static ergonomics are not sufficient for the right sitting. Dynamic ergonomics are required in light of the latest medical discoveries.

Static sitting ergonomics makes sure to support your right body posture. On the other hand, dynamic sitting ergonomics makes sure to accommodate the movement of your body, continuously supporting your posture, while your body moves and shifts from one position to another, keeping your trunk active, even gently stimulating the movement of your trunk as required.

Your sitting devices or back supports must be able to

accommodate, facilitate, even stimulate the movement of your trunk and pelvis. If your chairs, seats, or couches are too expansive to upgrade, you can choose the proper add-ons to them for this purpose.

Your seat or chair must be able to provide a dynamic sitting foundation to accommodate your body's need for motion. It also needs to be ergonomic to facilitate the right sitting posture and spinal alignment.

2. Compute Right

With regards to spinal health, the following are the six critical mistakes that computers users frequently make:

1. Slouched back,
2. Tilted head and neck,
3. Closed chest,
4. Lack of physical activity in the trunk for too long,
5. Poor alignment between the chair or the seat and the desk,
6. Poor position of the computer monitor.

Having the right understanding and using the right work station will go a long way to reduce or alleviate many of the above mentioned problems. The right workstation needs to be able to help you achieve the right alignment of your chair level and that of your desk, the right positioning of your computer monitor, the right alignment of your visual focus with the head posture, the right alignment of your work surface and your back posture.

Your work station is comprised of your seat, your desk, and your computer. Their heights and the distances between them need to be aligned properly. Proper alignment will allow your thighs to have a 90 to a 100 degree angle from your trunk when you sit upright with both of your feet resting on the ground comfortably. The right alignment should also allow your forearms comfortably resting on the desk with a 10 to a 20 degree angle between your upper arms and your trunk and a 90 to 100 degree angle between your forearm and upper arm, when sitting upright.

The right workstation also needs to allow your hands to be on or slightly below the extension line of your forearm. To make this happen, the simplest way is to rest your forearm on the edge of your desk with the edge touching the lower part of your forearm one to two inches from the tip of your elbow. Slightly drop your elbow and tilt your forearm slightly upwards while maintaining a angle of 90 to 100 degrees between your forearm and your upper arm. Such upward tilts of your forearm will allow sufficient space between your key board underneath your hands. You can then comfortably drop your fingers on the key board and type with your hands slightly tilted downwards.

The alignment between the various components of your workstation is far more critical than the quality of your seat, desk, and computer separately, because this alignment has a greater impact on your body mechanics. You can have a lousy and harmful workstation, if your chairs, desks, and computer are the best in the workplace separately, but are poorly aligned at an integrated workstation.

The seat is the foundation of your posture. The desk is the condition of your posture. And the computer screen is the guide of your posture. The miss-alignment of any one of these three key components is sufficient to lead to unexpected stress, and tension and suffering in your back, neck, hands, productivity, and wellbeing. Over time, the cumulative effect will be sufficient to lead to problems or even pain in your back. As a result, you need to adjust the alignment whenever you begin to use a new workstation for a prolonged period.

As discussed before, you must also keep movements in your trunk and back while sitting. You need to take frequent breaks for the neck and back movement, relaxation, and exercises. If you can't take frequent breaks, one of the most practical approaches is to sit with proprioceptive stimulation, which forces your body to balance itself continuously. In this process, your spine will move like a small tree in the wind – gently swinging back and forth, which activates the deep stabilizing muscles in your back and keeps them continuously engaged to stay in action.

Another critical mistake most computer users make is the poor alignment between their hands and their key boards. One of the most frequent health problems that happen to computer users is carpal tunnel syndrome. The key cause is repetitive strains in the wrist due to the upward bending of the hands. The right alignment of the hands to the arms while typing or using a mouse is that hands need to be in the same line as the arm or slightly dropped downwards from the extension line of the arm. Unfortunately, most computer desks, keyboards, and mice, no matter how expensive they are or how ergonomic they claim to be, tend to force the hand to tilt upwards from the extension line of the arm, which is a sure recipe for abnormal stress in the wrist and the eventual onset of carpal tunnel syndrome. Stressed wrists may lead to premature fatigue of the computer users, which can affect his/her back, head, neck, and chest posture negatively.

3. Lift Right

There are six major mistakes people make when lifting a heavy object:

- First, standing too far from the object and bending your body far out to reach it.

- Second, lifting the object without it touching your body, as if it was an infectious alien.

- Third, failing to take and holding a big breath while exerting the force during the lift.

- Fourth, failing to use the legs, instead of the spine.

- Fifth, lack of a proper plan when you have to lift a heavy object for a longer distance.

- Sixth, failing to do the above things before lifting a heavy object.

You must assure a right position of your body by standing as close to the object as possible. From a biomechanical point of view, you want to stand over the object, with it between your legs. The right position of your body allows the best possible exertion of your force, and often means half of the battle against the heavy object is won. Without positioning your body properly, the general wisdom of "keeping heavy objects close to the body" will become an empty phrase.

If at all possible, you want to have the heavy object touching your body (the abdomen or waist area). This assures that you are keeping heavy objects as close to your body as possible. Wear casual clothes that you will not regret if it becomes dirty or damaged. If this is not possible, grab a piece of cloth, a hand towel, a piece of cardboard, or a piece of paper, to protect your skin or nice clothes while you hold the object in-line with your body, while actually TOUCHING it. Letting your heavy object touching your body is critical, because it doesn't touch your body, you are not hold it close enough to your body, and your back suffers unnecessarily.

Taking and holding a big breath of air is one of the most important things to do, especially when the object is extra heavy. As discussed before, it dramatically increases the leaver length of your back muscles to make the force your back muscles exert often up to four times more effective. In other words, if you take and hold a big breath, you will be able to reduce the stress in your back muscles by up to three quarters, while lifting the same object, or you will be able to lift up to a four-times heavier object with the same level of stress in your back muscles.

To protect your back or to be able to life more weight, you must use your legs as much as possible. Many people keep their legs straight and bend their lower back to reach for a heavy object on the ground, and lift it up by straightening their back upwards. Such an approach is almost a sure recipe to injure the back.

The right way is to bend the legs, while keeping the back as straight and upright as possible, to reach the object, keep your chest open, and lift the object by pushing up with your legs. Please remember to bend your legs instead of your back while reaching out to the object, and straighten your legs not your back while lifting a heavy object, instead of the other way around, which is what most people do most time.

It will be too late to try to figure out your game plan to move a heavy object for a long distance when a heavy TV set is already in your hands, and your muscles are screaming from pain caused by the load. Ask any professional mover, and they will tell you that you have to plan in advance. You need to have the destination prepared, ready to accept the object. You need to plan the supporting or resting spots in between the origin and the destination of the object. You need to prepare the supporting spots, so that you don't have to lay the object all the way down to the ground and lift it all the way up again, because the putting down and lifting up process are the most energy consuming, technically complex, and bodily most risky activities of the whole lifting and moving process.

Last but not least, you must make sure you do the above preparatory activities, BEFORE you begin to lift it up. Needless to say, the heavier the object, the more important to do all the above activities right before your lifting activity.

If the object is extra heavy, you also want to flex up and warm up your body, before you begin. You may also consider using a back support belt.

If your profession requires you lift or move heavy objects on a regular basis, you need to seriously participate in back strengthening exercises, especially those exercises that help strengthen the deep stabilizing muscles in the back. Exercises with sitting on an unstable surface, such as Swiss Balls, air discs or pillows are all beneficial. (Note: Power bending will do little to strengthen these small deep stabilizing muscles.)

4. Read Right
Reading often leads to poor posture, both in the lower back and in the neck. While keeping your back straight, you must also keep your head and neck aligned with your back.

Your head needs to be kept in the extension line of your back as much as possible. It is important to reduce or prevent your head from tilting. The key is to keep your book or electronic reader up, ideally at your eye level. Your posture, not only your head but also, to a large extent, your back posture, is guided by your eyesight. Where your eyesight aims and how you use your eyesight often determines your posture.

The way you sit and position your body also determines your posture. If you sit upright and lean your upper body forward from your hip, instead of from your lower back or neck, you will be able to maintain a better posture for your back and neck.

If you sit and lean back on a couch, your head may be required to tilt forward to be able to read your book, unless you hold your book really high, which may be so tiring to your arms that it becomes unsustainable. In addition, sitting and leaning back on a couch often flattens your lower back and destroys the posture of your back.

If you need to read from a computer screen, you need to consider raising the computer screen to the level of your eyes.

In the case where it is not practical to position your book or reading screen in a right height, you may want to tilt your eyesight to reduce the tilt of your head and neck.

As a result, you have two measures to compensate the short comings of your seat or the position of your book or reading screen. First is your hip. Lean your body from your hip, instead of your lower back or your neck. Second is your eyesight. Tilt your eyesight instead of your head or neck.

5. Drive Right

Car seats are notoriously poorly designed for your back health. Most car seats, including those in the premium automobiles, will force your back into a forward bending "C" curve. Also most drivers, especially tall and young male drivers, tend to put the back of their seat into a reclined position. In order to watch the road traffic, they have to lift their head up from the head rest, and essentially put their head and neck in a forward head posture. While it may be a cool style of driving, such posture would most frequently lead to stiffness, pain or fatigue in the neck, headache, and other complications on long trips.

It is important to use a proper back support to protect your lower back curvature and keep motion in your back on long rides. It is important to realize that the support in most premium automobiles is not up to the job. It is also important to keep the back of your seat upright instead of in a reclined position. This is not only good for relieving the stress in your neck, but also good for your safety in the case of an auto accident.

Head up. Back straight. Seat back upright at a 95 to 100 degree recline.

The JazzRX is specially engineered for long distance trips. Proven by independent clinical study to help 86 percent back sufferers relieve back pain.

6. Game Right

There are three frequently occurring problems with electronic gaming:

- Forward tilted head and neck,
- Flattened lower back, and
- Closed chest.

Forward tilted head and neck often lead to Forward Head Posture, a nagging, sometimes, debilitating pain in the neck and upper back. It can cause persistent headaches, premature degeneration of the cervical spine, and a plain poor look and indigent personal image, over time.

A flattened lower back often dramatically increases the stress, tension, and pressure in the lower back muscles and the discs, and is a key factor for stiff and sore backs.

Closed chest, or Forward Rolling Shoulders, not only leads to a poor look and personal image that no amount of expensive cosmetics can mask, but also compromises the vital capacity and increases the risk of forward head posture.

Whether you are sitting or standing while gaming on your electronic devices, you must pay attention to keep your head and neck aligned with your back and spine, to reduce, and prevent your head from tilting forward, as much as possible. You must keep your back straight and prevent your lower back from being flattened. And you must keep your chest open at all times.

Taking frequent breaks is tremendously helpful in allowing your body to resume a healthy posture.

Having your monitor properly aligned with your chair and seat is essential for you to maintain a healthy posture.

For more details, please refer to the above discussion on "Read Right."

7. Sleep Right

To sleep right, you must also use the right sleeping pillow. This is particularly important because 98 percent of all sleeping pillows are designed incorrectly and function poorly.

It is a myth that back sleepers should use a pillow to prop up the thighs. What is critical to back sleepers is to use a proper device to prop up their lower back to protect their lumbar curvature. Propping up the thighs tend to flatten out the lumbar curvature, worsen the spinal mechanics, and increases the stress and tension in the back that can lead to morning back pain. The world renowned "back doctor"

Dr. Hamilton Hall, suggests that patients use a proper support to the lordosis while sleeping.

Certainly propping up the thighs can feel comfortable to many people. Without supporting the lower back, the benefit of propping the thighs is limited.

First of all, most pillows lack cervical support. A healthy neck is arched and is smaller in diameter than the head. Without proper cervical support, the neck will be forced to bend unnaturally or lose its natural alignment and curvature, which causes your neck ligaments and muscles to be ill-stretched, and often leads to neck pain.

Second, most sleeping pillows are too thick in the area that supports the back of your head when sleeping on your back. Sleeping pillow manufacturers seem to lack an understanding about why a sleeping pillow is needed, and what determines the right height of the sleeping pillow. Essentially a sleeping pillow is required to maintain a spinal alignment that is natural to a person when she or he stands upright comfortably. To a person with a healthy neck posture and curvature, the compressed height of the sleeping pillow should be roughly the distance in the back of the person's head where it protrudes from his back horizontally, which is mostly between zero and one inch. As a result, the area of the pillow that is designed to support the back of a head should be no more than one inch in thickness. Yet, the corresponding thickness of most sleeping pillows are three inches or more, which pushes the head into a forward translated position and helps to cement the forward head posture into a clinical condition over time.

Third, the area designed to support the head when sleeping on a side is frequently too thick. Sleeping pillow manufacturers often provide the pillow thickness to fit the distance between your ear to the end of your shoulder. However, your shoulders tend to curl up due to your body weight when you roll to the side. The required height of supporting your head to maintain a reasonable alignment with your spine is often reduced by 50 percent.

Fourth, the rear end of most sleeping pillows is too thick, even if the area that supports the back of the head is thin enough. Most pillows intend to make the rear end of the pillow to be suitable for cervical support but with a different thickness compared to the cervical support at the front end of the pillow, in order to suit individuals of different body sizes. The sad reality is that, due to the limited depth of the pillow, the thick part at the rear end often interferes with the head by pushing it up or by turning the head slightly forward, even if ever so slightly. The interference creates unnecessary pressure and stress in the neck and compromises the quality of sleep, even causes neck pain in the morning.

As a result, finding a pillow that doesn't have most of any of the above four issues will go a long way in helping your neck and sleep.

Use the right pillow: neck support is a must; thickness underneath the back of your head < 1.5 inch, after weight loading; thickness underneath the side of your head equals half of the horizontal distance between the outer edge of your shoulder and your ear.

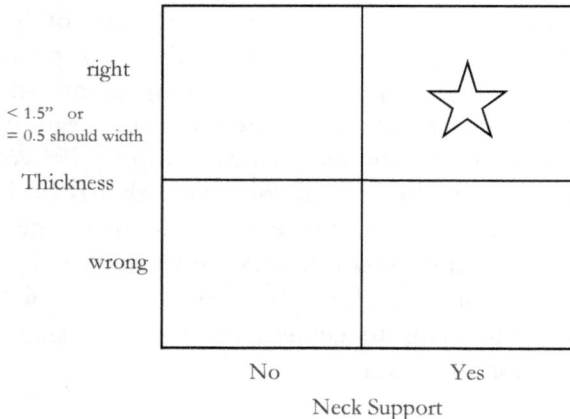

Source: Patrick Lee

Fig. 3.9

The right pillow should not push your head into a forward head posture while sleeping on your back, and should not make your head tilt up or downwards so much that your head is significantly out of the extension line of your spine.

Use the right mattress: your bed should not be like a hammock. Hammocks may appear to be cozy and romantic for a tropical island vacation. It is not good for your back, because it causes your back to lose its lordosis (curvature) when you sleep on your back or causes your back to curl like a fish, both of which worsen the biomechanical condition of your spine and raise the stress and tension to your spinal discs and soft tissues although you do not realize it.

Firmer mattresses are better. Your mattress must be firm enough to keep the spine leveled and straight, no hammock syndrome.

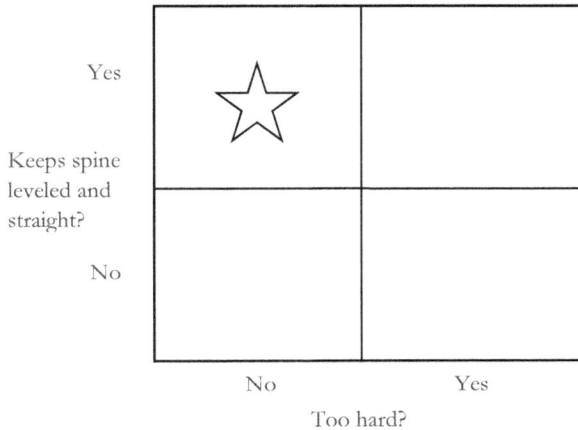

Source: Patrick Lee

Fig. 3.10

Don't worry too much about your "comfort" when making habitual changes to your body. There will be no change in your bodily habit, if there is no short-term discomfort. Your body's current sense of sleeping comfort may be the result of a bad habit which contributed to your back problem in the first place. To resolve your back problems, you must first resolve the bad habit. You will feel "uncomfortable" during the initial phase of correction. Your body will naturally adapt to your new healthy mattress and pillow, and appreciate them in time.

8. Stand Right

Prolonged standing has long been linked to lower back pain, because of two reasons:

First, during prolonged still standing, like during prolonged still sitting, the deep stabilizing muscles in the back will tend to tense. In a recent study from McGill University in Canada, researchers asked eighteen participants to stand upright, as the stiffness of their back muscles as well as the blood flow in their lower body were monitored. After only 25-minutes all participant were experiencing muscular stiffness in their lower back, with some stiffness starting as soon as the standing began, according to Dr. Julie Cote, an Associate Professor of Biomechanics and Ergonomics at the university. The study also found that minimal to no circulation of blood (blood pooling), in the participants' legs after just 15-minutes of standing.

Second, prolonged standing often leads to poor standing posture and biomechanics to the spine. People's waist tends to gradually shift forward, pelvis tilts forward, upper body sways backwards and slumps, and head leans forward. In this process, the extra pull on the ligaments and muscles and increased pressure and stress in the spine could cause aches, pains, stiffness, and fatigue in the back.

Therefore, it is important to prevent the stillness while you stand. Keep motion in your back and legs while keeping an upright posture. From the side view, a finger width distance forward of your ear, the center of your shoulder, the center of your pelvis and the center of your ankle should be aligned in one gravity line (your body's natural state of balance).

Make sure you stand in good body biomechanics:

- Stand on even ground,
- Head and back upright,
- Chest open,
- Muscles comfortably relaxed,
- Eyes forward horizontally,
- Head, trunk and legs aligned in one gravity line.

Make sure you stand in good biomechanics and make sure you give yourself a good standing foundation. There are many anti-fatigue standing mats on the market. The better ones are made of Polyurethane material and are capable of stimulating your body with a continued gentle instability to help you gently shift your standing posture, improve blood circulation, and reduce muscle tension. When you are standing, the best posture is always the next one. A dynamic posture that constantly and gently shifts is the key to prevent fatigue.

Find opportunities to reduce standing. Often your standing can be relieved by using a high chair which will keep you high up but significantly relieve the strain on your legs. Better high chairs are those that are dynamic with the seats moving with your body and buttocks to help you prevent still sitting. Whether you work in a retail store, or mind a tradeshow booth, or are working in an office, using a high chair is almost always a practical option.

Also find opportunities to walk around a little bit. This is possible in most situations. Our body is not built for sitting. Moving around helps relax your muscles and gives them a chance to recuperate from its tensions.

9. Walk Right

Keep your upper body upright, and minimize the forward bending of your back or neck, and look forward well ahead, instead of just a few feet ahead of your toes. To facilitate your walking, you may shift your upper body slightly forward from your hips, while keeping your spine straight.

The distance between your feet should be roughly the width of your hips. It is already too wide if it equals your shoulder width.

It is better to walk at a brisk pace – comfortably fast. Slow walking creates more constant pressure and stress on your back, that are harder to recover from.

Try to keep your pelvis relatively stable instead of letting it swing back and forth with each step forward.

Push your pelvis forward with your hind leg, instead of pulling your pelvis forward with your front leg. As a general principle of using your body correctly, pushing is preferred over pulling.

Gently swing your arms as you take each step. Proper arm movements facilitate smooth hip rotation, and ease of alternative stepping. Fixed arms increase the stress and tension in the back. Take your hands out of your pockets and let your arms move naturally.

In order to walk right, you need to use the right shoes. Unfortunately, high heels and loose slippers are not among the right shoes. From a health and biomechanics point of view, human shoes do not need heels, and there is no such thing as a "perfect walk in high heels." It is a myth that shoes should have heels.

Biomechanically speaking, a heel on a shoe causes the thigh to shift forward and the pelvis tilts forward, which inevitably forces the upper body to sway backwards to balance the posture, and the backward swayed upper body in turn forces the head and neck to lean forward. This chain effect is true when you stand still, but also true when you walk. And when you run, the heels effectively turn themselves into health and safety hazards. None of these effects of the heel is good for the human body in any way.

Uneven heels and blown out heels destroy your healthy body balance, body biomechanics, postural alignment, and gait. Men are often guilty of wearing shoes with blown out heels that are worn down on one side completely. Your shoes are not just there to protect your skin from the hazard on the road. Your shoes are there to support your posture and gait. Poor heels lead to poor posture and gait. The money saved by wearing out a pair of shoes with blown out heels will be surpassed 10,000 times by the cost of recovering your back from injury, dysfunction or pain, in due time. Think of your shoes as an investment for the health of your spine, instead of consumables for protection of the skin on your feet.

Your spine is the equivalent of the transmission of your car. Without a properly functioning transmission, your car will not be able to go anywhere. Should your car start to stand up right, the tires of your car would also be your investment in maintaining your transmission, instead of for your wheels only.

Try to select a pair of shoes with the lowest heel possible that you enjoy wearing. Repair the heels of your shoes timely to prevent severely worn heels. Your back will thank you for your wise decision.

10. Garden Right
Gardening is an activity that often leads to sore or stiff backs and necks.

The key problems with gardening are two folds:
- Forward tilting of the neck, and
- Forward bending of the back.

The first secret for combating these problems, is your knowledge about what of the gardening activities creates sore backs and sore necks.

The second is to consciously maintain a good posture and prevent the forward tilting of the neck and the forward bending of the back.

The third secret is to use a kneeling pad or a knee pad. Such pads will give the critical support that your body needs, and help you better maintain a good posture for your back and neck.

The forth secret is to use tools with long handles. Long handles allows you to reduce the forward tilting and bending. A few more dollars spent on the right tools with the right handles will save you hundredfold, if not thousand fold, in terms of money and time from treating your back and neck pain down the road.

Keep your back straight. Move your upper body forward and backward from your hips with the control of your legs, instead of from the middle of your lower back. Keep your neck straight as much as you can. If you do need to get your eyes closer to the work you are doing, rotate your upper body forward from the hips instead of leaning your head forward in a similar fashion as you protect your back.

Use your legs to lower your body and hands, instead of bending your back for the same purpose.

11. Shovel Right

Snow shoveling is literally a breath-taking activity. It is not only labor and energy intensive and often takes your breath away, but also tends to force your body into a poor posture and leads to back pain. In the Northern regions of the USA and Canada, snow shoveling tends to be a leading cause for back injuries and pain in the winter season.

It is important to maintain a good posture while shoveling. Keep your back as straight as possible. Bend your body forward from the hips instead of from your lower back. Use your legs and arms instead of your back.

Use a snow plow and thrower if you can. A few hundred dollars of investment in one of these machines will save you thousands of dollars of expenditure on your doctor's visits and medical treatments for your back pain down the road. Considering your financial investments, there would be few investment opportunities that could ever bring you a return remotely as high as the above investment.

Use a shovel with a long handle. Short handles will force your body to lean forward, especially if you are a tall person.

Use a shovel with a special ergonomic curve in its handle designed to reduce the forward leaning of your upper body.

Take frequent breaks. Don't try to finish shoveling your drive way in one go. The fresh air and deep temperatures tantalizes you to keep going with your shoveling, even when your deep back muscles already start to fatigue. Take a break every 10-minutes. Stop for two-minutes before resuming shoveling. In the breaks, walk around a bit.

Stretch your back a little. Shake your arms and legs a few times. All these will help you recover from the stress and regain your body's readiness for further shoveling.

Your muscles need time to recuperate from stresses put on them. In such cases, while the stress is not sufficient to break them right away, the cumulative effect of the repetitive application of the stress is what may hurt your back. This represents one kind of repetitive strain injury.

12. Regular Checks and Care Like You Do For Your Teeth

Take care of your spine and back in the same way you do for your teeth. Your spine is far more important than your teeth, and deserves at least the equal care, attention, and investment compared to your teeth. See your doctor for your spine on a regular basis, as you do with your dentist. By the way, dentists have one of the highest rates of back pain among all healthcare professionals.

Too often in today's society, behind a mouthful of beautiful teeth is a suffering spine and a painful back. This compromises your energy to smile and show off your beautiful teeth That compromises your mobility to move around, including your favorite restaurants to use your beautiful teeth at, while further compromising your mood and spirit to even feel, notice or enjoy your beautiful teeth.

Take care of your spine and back in the same way as you do for your teeth. You will thank yourself when you see those who don't suffer down the road. Ignore this advice at your own peril.

4

6 Secret Nutritional Foods Your Body Cries For

The right food and diet may not relieve your pain overnight. However, it may be indispensable in your fight against spinal illness. The right food and diet will help you:

- Better rebuild ligaments and muscles to recover from injuries,
- Better maintain the health of your spinal joints to reduce or prevent spinal degeneration,
- Better maintain the health of your vertebral bones, bone mass and bone marrow to prevent vertebral facture and prevent back pain,
- Better hydrate your spinal discs to slow down degeneration in your body, and
- Better maintain a favorable environment in your body to fight inflammation.

1. Tart Cherries

A research paper presented by Dr. Kerry Kuehl of Oregon Health & Science University, at the American College of Sports Medicine

Conference (ACSM) in San Francisco, California in 2012, found that tart cherries have the highest anti-inflammatory content of any food, "…and may help reduce chronic inflammation among those suffering joint pain and arthritis."

The study involved twenty women ages 40 to 70 with inflammatory osteoarthritis, and found that drinking tart cherry juice twice daily for three weeks resulted in significant reductions in important inflammation markers – especially among women who had the highest inflammation levels at the start of the study.

"With millions of Americans looking for ways to naturally manage pain, it's promising that tart cherries can help, without the possible side effects often associated with arthritis medications," said Dr. Kerry Kuehl. "I'm intrigued by the potential for a real food to offer such a powerful anti-inflammatory benefit – especially for active adults."

Dr. Kuehl's findings may also be highly beneficial to athletes. In a past study, he found that people who drank tart cherry juice, while training for a long distance run, reported significantly less pain after exercise than those who didn't.

The pigment that gives tart cherry its color is called anthocyanin. Anthocyanins are water-soluble vacuolar pigments that may appear red, purple, or blue depending on the pH level. Natural anthocyanin food color pigments have been proven to have strong antioxidant and anti-inflammatory properties. This may also be the reason why red, purple, and black foods, such as beets, purple sweet potatoes, and red wine, are often excellent anti-oxidant and anti-inflammatory foods, but only if you also eat their skin because often the anthocyanin is mainly contained in the skin of the food. Once peeled their health properties reduce dramatically. Of course foods such as beets are different from foods such as cherries, because their flesh is also purple. But still, their skins tend to have the highest concentration of anthocyanin.

2. Ginger

The anti-inflammatory properties of ginger have been known and valued for thousands of years. It has a long history of being used as medicine in Asian and Arabic herbal traditions. In China, for example, ginger has been used to treat cold, flu, digestion, stomach upset, and diarrhea for more than 2,000 years.

According to Grzanna R, Lindmark L, Frondoza CG, ginger's anti-inflammatory properties have been repeatedly proven and confirmed by various studies since these properties were first confirmed and ginger was formally defined as a herbal medical product in the west in the early 1970s. The initial discovery revealed that ginger shares pharmacological properties with non-steroidal anti-inflammatory drugs (NSAID, such as ibuprofen-based Advil).

"An important extension of this early work was the observation that ginger also suppresses leukotriene biosynthesis by inhibiting 5-lipoxygenase," the study says. "This pharmacological property distinguishes ginger from nonsteroidal anti-inflammatory drugs. This discovery preceded the observation that dual inhibitors of cyclooxygenase and 5-lipoxygenase may have a better therapeutic profile and have fewer side effects than non-steroidal anti-inflammatory drugs."

"The characterization of the pharmacological properties of ginger entered a new phase with the discovery that a ginger extract (EV.EXT.77) derived from Zingiber officinale (family Zingiberaceae) and Alpina galanga (family Zingiberaceae) inhibits the induction of several genes involved in the inflammatory response. These include genes encoding cytokines, chemokines, and the inducible enzyme cyclooxygenase-2. This discovery provided the first evidence that ginger modulates biochemical pathways activated in chronic inflammation. Identification of the molecular targets of individual ginger constituents provides an opportunity to optimize and standardize ginger products with respect to their effects on specific biomarkers of inflammation."

In plain language, ginger may be more effective than NSAIDs and have far less side effects than NSAIDs. Ginger may be especially beneficial to sufferers with chronic back pain. It may take several weeks for ginger to start helping reduce pain.

3. Garlic

Garlic has been regarded as medicinal food since ancient times, and can be used in many ways, for a wide range of health conditions. It is a miracle food.

Garlic is rich in antioxidants. Your immune system could benefit if you give it a constant boost of powerful garlic in daily recipes. Try garlic in your cooking, add garlic to your sauces, drink garlic tea with sliced or minced garlic steeped in hot water.

Its antioxidants kill bacteria, so rub a sliced clove of garlic on a pimple for an effective topical treatment. It has been widely used to treat acne, colds, athlete's foot, psoriasis, and cold sores.

4. Fatty Ocean Fish, Such as Wild Salmon, Herring, and Sardines

Fatty ocean fish are rich in Omega 3 that has long been associated with powerful anti-inflammatory benefits. The mechanism behind this link was revealed in a 2010 study published in *Cell*. This study identified that G protein-coupled receptor 120 (GPR120) protein functions as an Omega-3 FA sensor. Stimulation of GPR120 protein with Omega-3 FAs creates broad anti-inflammatory effects in cells. Consuming fatty ocean fish, such as salmon, herring, and sardines, can help stimulate the anti-inflammatory reactions in cells and help control back pain involving inflammation.

However, the fish need to be prepared in a healthy way. A 2009 study from the University of Hawaii found that men who ate baked or boiled fish (i.e. cooked fresh with low fat, not cooked in less healthy ways, such as fried, dried, or salted) cut their risk of heart disease by 23 percent.

5. Purple Sweet Potatoes

There are over 400 kinds of sweet potatoes. They differ in skin and flesh color from white to purple.

Purple sweet potatoes may be one of the world's healthiest foods. And it is the secret nutrition source of my friend Mr. Lee Haney – an eight time Mr. Olympia -- one the most successful body builders the world has ever seen. He lives on purple sweet potatoes. And he must know what he is doing.

Purple sweet potato color extracted from purple sweet potatoes has been proven to be able to attenuate or constrict the oxidative degradation of the vital building blocks of living cells (called lipids), renew the activities of antioxidant enzymes and suppress inflammatory responses in the body.

According to some studies, the antioxidant density of purple sweet potatoes is three-times as high as that of blueberries.

Purple sweet potatoes are richer in vitamin A than most green leafy vegetables. The only food that is richer in vitamin A is beef liver. It is also rich in vitamin C and B6.

6. Water

Most of our body consists of water. A plentiful supply of water helps the body transport nutrients and remove waste. Proper hydration of the body is critical for soft tissue recovery and regeneration, as well as for proper hydration of the spinal discs.

Dehydration can lead to muscle spasms, kidney problems, and other conditions that can cause pain in the back.

According to The Institute of Medicine, an adequate intake of total liquid for an average man is roughly 3.7 liters a day, and for a woman it is 2.7 liters. This total amount includes the liquid contained in all your daily food and beverage intake. About 20 percent of your liquid intake is from your food.

For your convenience, simply remember to drink 8 x 8 water --. 8 glasses of 8 ounces of water a day. This is not completely in line with the advice of the Institute of Medicine, but is generally more than the amount most people drink guided by their thirst each day. Drink more if you need to, especially in hot weather or when participating in physically intensive sports or work, or when you are breast feeding, or if you have fever or diarrhea.

Of course, your water intake requirements also depends on your body weight. For a more accurate amount for your particular situation, you may want to take advantage of the water intake calculator at about.com:

http://nutrition.about.com/library/blwatercalculator.htm

7. Other Foods

There are many other foods that are effective in helping your body manage inflammation, oxidation, aging, and the degeneration processes, hence good for your back and spinal health. Your body needs a wide range of critical nutrients. Any food rich in the following elements are desirable for you. Consume such foods purposefully.

a. Vitamin B12

Vitamin B12 is critical to keep the body producing its own most important antioxidant glutathione. It also helps keep the body's nerve and blood cells healthy and helps make DNA, while often used to boost energy. A 2000 study found that taking vitamin B12 may help relieve back pain.

According to the Office of Dietary Supplements of the National Institutes of Health, foods that are rich in vitamin B12 include beef liver, clams, wild trout, and salmon.

b. Vitamin D

Vitamin D helps with calcium absorption and building strong bones, which is essential in preventing osteoporosis. It can also help alleviate back pain by reducing inflammation. Vitamin D deficiency is linked with osteomalacia, a disease in which adults experience softening of the bones, causing bending of the spine, bowing of the legs, bone fragility, and increased risk for fractures.

Vitamin D can be found in fatty fish, such as salmon and mackerel. As the sunshine vitamin, the easiest way to obtain Vitamin D is to go out and bath in natural sunlight.

c. Vitamin K

Vitamin K is critical for the bones to properly use calcium. The combination of vitamin K and calcium help bones stay strong and healthy. Deficiency in vitamin K may increase the risk of osteoporosis and arthritis.

Typical natural foods rich in vitamin K are green vegetables, including kale, spinach, mustard greens, collard greens, Swiss chard, turnip greens, parsley, broccoli, and Brussels sprouts.

d. Calcium

Calcium is essential for bone health and bone mass. It is important in preventing osteoporosis, which often results in vertebral fractures, spinal deformation, and back pain.

Calcium is rich in dairy products, such as milk, yogurt, and cheese. It is also rich in dark green vegetables, such as spinach, broccoli, and kale. Soy and soy products, such as tofu and soy milk, are also rich in calcium. Fatty fish, such as salmon and sardines, are also an excellent source for calcium.

e. Iron

Iron is important for cells to remain healthy and maintain the health of muscles that are critical to support a healthy spine.

Iron is rich in meat products, such as liver, red meat, port, poultry, eggs, fish, and shellfish. It is also rich in lentils, beans, soy, grains, and green leafy vegetables, such as spinach, kale, and broccoli.

f. Magnesium

Magnesium is critical in calcium metabolism and hormone production, that regulates the calcium. Both calcium metabolism and hormone production are keys in promoting bone health, maintaining bone density, and protecting the spine against osteoporosis. Magnesium is also important for the relaxing and contracting of muscles. It helps muscles to maintain their tone.

Magnesium is rich in many natural foods. Top magnesium rich foods include:

- Dark leafy vegetables, such as spinach, Swiss chard, and kale;
- Nuts and seeds, such as squash and pumpkin seeds, brazil nuts, almonds, cashews and pine nuts;
- Some fish including mackerel, Pollock, turbot, and tuna;
- Beans and lentils including soy, white beans, French beans, black-eyed peas, and kidney beans;
- Whole grains, such as brown rice, quinoa, millet, bulgur, buckwheat, and wild rice;
- Avocado;
- Low fat dairy, such as hard goat cheese, and nonfat yogurt;
- Bananas, and dried fruits, such as figs, prunes, apricots;
- And dark chocolate.

g. Antioxidants

An antioxidant is a molecule that removes free radicals and protects other molecules from oxidation, which can cause damage or death to the cells. Antioxidants are important in helping the immune system keep inflammation low and fight off diseases, slows down the aging process and maintaining the general health of the body. Antioxidants are important in helping the body fight inflammation and repair tissues, and are important to help reduce back pain that involves inflammation.

Our body produces a number of antioxidants by itself, including glutathion, vitamin C, vitamin A, and vitamin E, as well as various enzymes, such as catalase, superoxide dismutase, and various peroxidases.

Glutathion may be the most powerful antioxidant because it is produced by the body itself and used for the most critical defense against toxins, and it also recycles itself. Once oxidized, glutathione can be regenerated back by glutathione reductase.

Unfortunately, most chronic diseases deplete glutathione and are associated with low levels of glutathione. According to Yale University Prevention Research Center, if you experience chronic illness or fatigue, low glutathione levels may be both the cause and result of the condition. You may want to have your doctor check it.

Vitamin C is critical for inflammation management and for the process that allows cells to be able to form into tissues, which is important for healing problems caused by injured soft tissues. It also keeps your immune system strong and accelerates the healing process. Vitamin C is rich in kiwis, oranges, grapefruits, strawberries, tomatoes, broccoli, spinach, red pepper, and sweet potatoes.

Vitamin A assists the immune system in fighting off diseases. It helps repair tissues and helps in the formation of bone. It also helps the body better use protein. Vitamin A is rich in beef, calf, and chicken liver, milk, cheese, eggs; apricots, nectarines, orange or green vegetables, such as carrots, sweet potatoes and spinach.

Vitamin E may help ease back pain helping your body to repair damaged tissue. As an antioxidant, it also boosts the immune system, improves circulation, and aids in the healing process. Foods rich with vitamin E include sunflower seeds and almonds.

There are many natural foods that contain high levels of antioxidants. It is recommendable to make them part of your regular diet.

5

8 Arts of Exercises You Need to Engage In

Exercises and your physical fitness are critical to both back pain relief and back pain prevention.

"Probably the best tool to minimize how frequently your back pain is going to reoccur is how fit you are," said Dr. Randy A. Shelerund, MD, Director of Spine Center, Mayo Clinic. "Your fitness drives how frequently your back pain will reoccur and how severe those reoccurrences will be."

A 2013 Consumer Report survey of 14,000 participants found that 58 percent of back pain sufferers, who had an episode in the past 12-months, wished they had done more exercises to strengthen their backs. Don't regret it when it is too late. Start exercise proactively. Start exercises now. Just do it.

No need to be a perfectionistic in selecting the ultimate form of exercises to do. If you don't have current acute back pain, any exercise is better than no exercise. Start with some of the simple exercises below to keep you going, and over time, you may wish to explore other great forms of exercises, such as Pilates, the Alexander

Technique, Yoga, Tai Chi and so on.

1. 33 #MadBack relief and preventative exercises on a stable surface

Regular exercises to restore the strength of your back and a gradual return to everyday activities are important for your full recovery. You may conduct some of the following exercises 10 to 30-minutes a day one to three-times a day during your early recovery. However, your exercise program should be supervised by your therapist or doctor.

It is important not to overdo yourself. You must progress gradually. Take on one exercise at a time. Starting from the most gentle ones.

If any exercise gives you any sharp pain in the back or legs, stop it immediately, and switch to another one. Sharp pains are often related to exaggeration of a fresh wound and pinched nerve. Little or no benefit could be gained by exaggerating a wound or pinching a nerve unnecessarily.

If any exercise gives you any deeper pain (instead of the muscle sore that one often gets after a good session of working out) that remains severe after a night of sleep, you also want to stop doing it.

Gently exercising and challenging your body is good to your recovery. Severely afflicting pain may deliver opposite results.

Above principles apply not only to patients with acute back pain but also to patients with chronic back pain.

If you don't have any back pain and simply want to do something to prevent it, you shouldn't experience any sharp or deep pain in the back or legs. However, you still need to begin with the most gentle ones first and take on only one new exercise each day. And always practice the general precautions for your exercises.

Consult a qualified advisor in case of any questions.

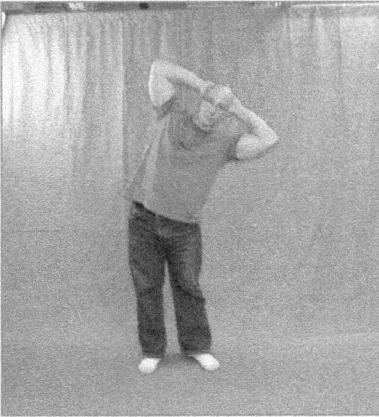

Exercise 1 (Standing Side-to-Side Shifts)
- Bend your arms behind your head.
- Gently bend your body towards the left.
- Gently return to a neutral position.
- Gently continue to bend towards the right.
- Gently return to a neutral position.
- Meanwhile face forward and keep your pelvis horizontal.
- 20 repetitions a day.

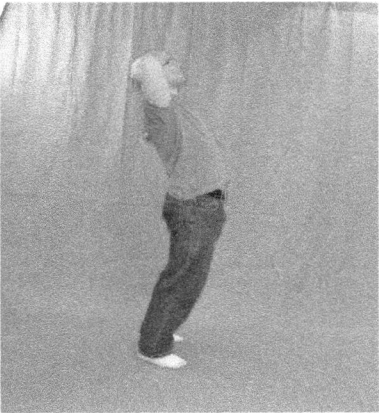

Exercise 2 (Standing Front to Back Tilts)
- Bend your arms behind your head.
- Gently bend your body backwards.
- Gently return to a neutral position.
- Gently continue to bend forward.
- Gently return to a neutral position.
- Meanwhile keep your legs and pelvis stable.
- 20 repetitions a day.

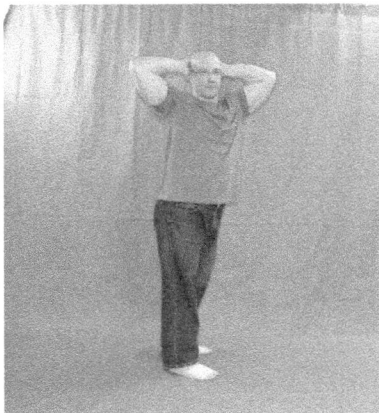

Exercise 3 (Standing Side to Side Rotations)
- Bend your arms behind your head.
- Gently rotate your body towards the right.
- Gently return to a neutral position.
- Gently continue to rotate your body towards left.
- Gently return to a neutral position.
- Meanwhile keep your legs and pelvis stable.
- 20 repetitions a day.

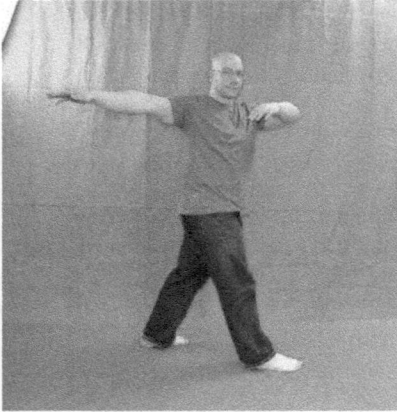

Exercise 4 (Walking Side to Side Rotations)

- Walk in large steps straight forward.
- Gently swing arms and the upper body in opposite directions of the forward foot.
- Gently swing upper body and arms to right when left foot moves forward.
- Gently return to a neutral position.
- Gently continue to swing upper body and arms to the left when right foot moves forward.
- Gently return to a neutral position.
- Walk 100 steps this way each day.

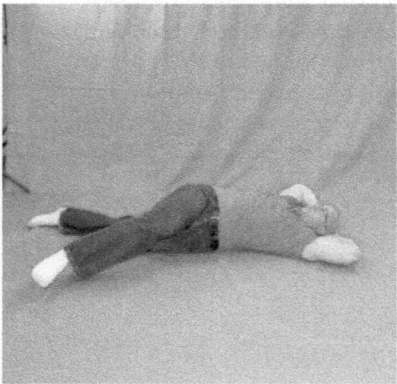

Exercise 5 (Lying Side to Side Rotations)

- Gently lie down on your back on the floor.
- Bend your arms behind your head.
- Gently raise your right foot and leg straight up.
- Gently turn your raised right foot and leg to the left.
- Gently continue to reach out to the left with the tip of your right foot, as much as you can.
- Gently return to a neutral position while keeping your right leg raised.
- Gently lower your right leg and foot to the floor.
- Repeat same motion with left leg and foot.
- 20 repetitions a day.

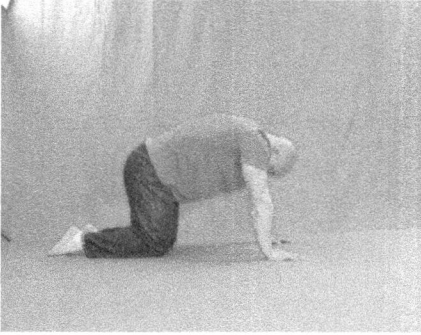

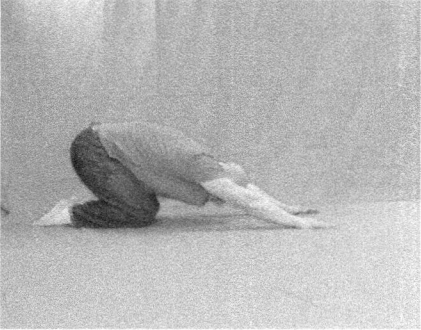

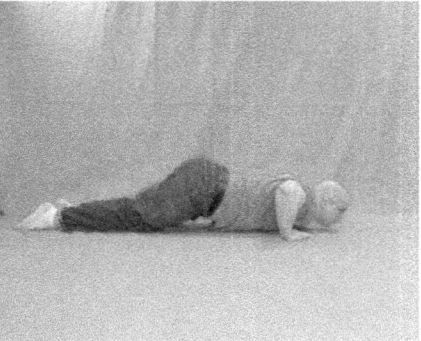

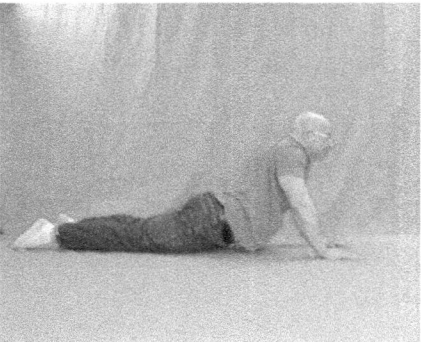

Exercise 6 (Lying Cat Stretch)

- Kneel on all fours while keeping your torso straight and your head aligned with your spine.
- Lift your lower and mid back as high as you can, like a cat, to make your back to form an arc.
- Gently shift your torso backward while keeping your lower and mid back lifted up as much as you can.
- Gently lower your shoulders while still keeping your lower and mid back lifted up as much as you can, like a cat stretches herself. Don't lift your head, continue to keep your head aligned with your spine.
- Gently move your torso forward while keeping your shoulders and body as low as you can without touching the floor, as if you were creeping forward and don't want to be detected, again like a cat.
- When your shoulders reach the position directly above your hands, you start to slowly push up your body with your arms. However, your torso may continue to move forward to its maximum. In this process, your head moves as if continuously pulled by the mid day sun and along a "c" curve that opens upward.
- When your arms stretch to their fullest, you begin to lift your waist and slowly move your torso backward. Try to lift your lower and mid back as high as possible, to make your back form an arc.
- 20 repetitions each day.

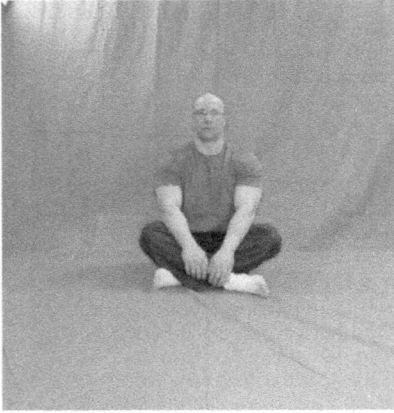

Exercise 7 (Seated Cross Body Reach)

- Sit on the floor with legs crossed.
- Gently raise your right knee and point your right foot forward.
- Gently pull your left leg to the right while keeping it close to you.
- Gently extend your left arm towards your right and past your right knee.
- Continue gently rotating your torso towards the right to the maximum you can. (well practiced individuals are able to rotate the torso until the left shoulder passes your raised right knee.)
- Hold for 5-seconds by counting the numbers 2001 and 2002, 2003 and 2004.
- Very gently and slowly return to a neutral position with legs crossed.
- Continue in the reversed direction.
- Gently raise your left knee and point your left foot forward.
- Gently pull your right leg to the left while keeping it close to you.
- Gently extend your right arm towards your left and past your left knee.
- Continue gently rotating your torso towards the left to the maximum you can. (well practiced individuals are able to rotate the torso until the right shoulder passes your raised left knee.)
- Hold for 5-seconds by counting the numbers 2001 and 2002, 2003, and 2004.
- Very gently and slowly return to a neutral position with your legs crossed.
- 10 repetitions each day.

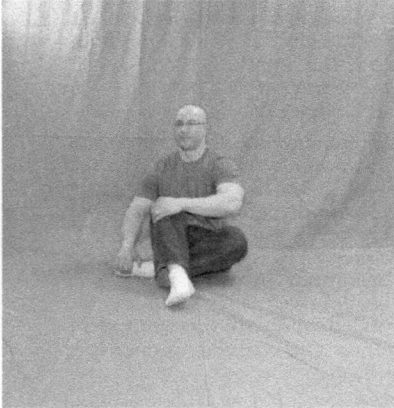

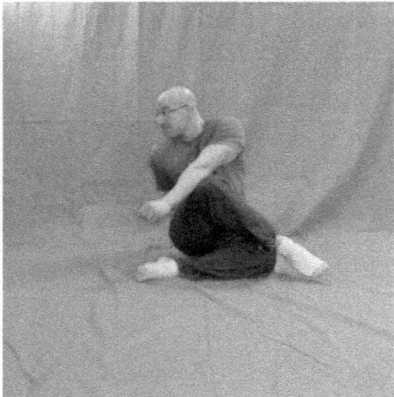

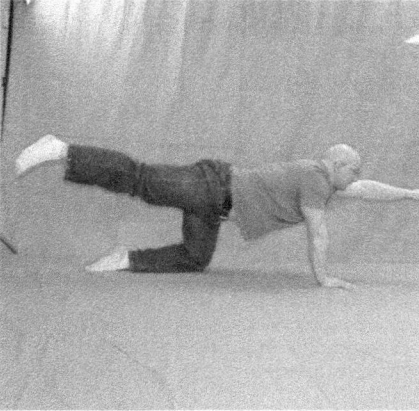

Exercise 8 (Kneeling Arm Reach)
- Kneel on all fours, while keeping your torso straight and your head aligned with your spine.
- Gently extend your left arm forward and extend your right leg backward, while maintaining your body balance with your right hand and left knee on the floor.
- Gently return to the neutral position of being on all fours.
- Repeat same motion with extending right arm and left leg.
- 20 repetitions a day.

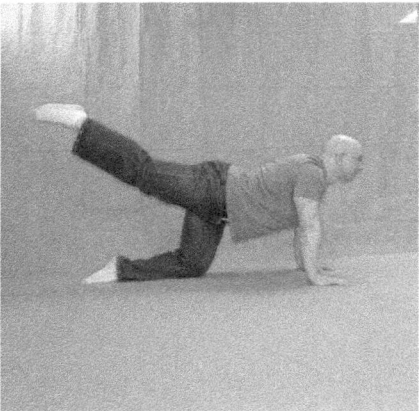

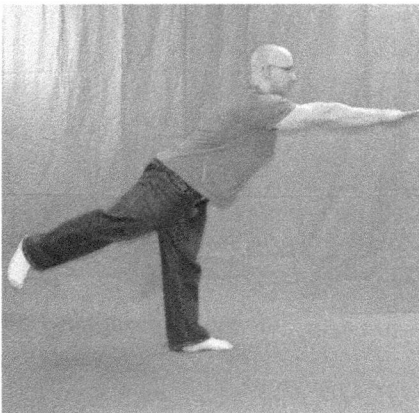

Exercise 9 (Knelling Leg Lift)
- Kneel on all fours, while keeping your torso straight and your head aligned with your spine.
- Gently extend your right leg backward while maintaining your body balance with your two hands and left knee on the floor.
- Gently return to the neutral position of being on all fours.
- Repeat same motion with extending left leg.
- 20 repetitions a day.

Exercise 10 (Standing Backward Leg Lift)
- Stand up straight.
- Gently extend both of your hands and arms forward.
- Gently lift your right leg backward, while maintaining your body balance on your left foot on the floor.
- Gently return to the neutral position of standing up straight.
- Repeat same motion with lifting your left leg backward, while maintaining your body balance on your right foot on the floor.
- 20 repetitions a day.

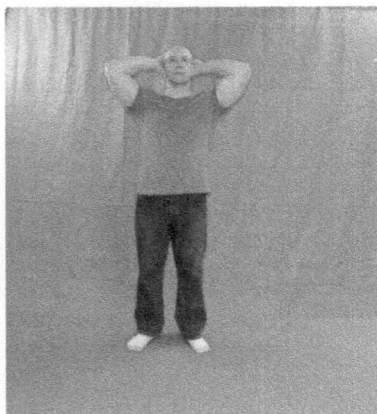

Exercise 11 (Standing Torso Rotations)

- Stand upright.
- Bend your arms behind your head.
- Gently rotate your torso clockwise first towards your right, then your front, then your left, and then your rear.
- Gently return to your neutral position of standing upright.
- Gently rotate your torso counter-clockwise first towards your left, then your front, then your right, then your rear.
- Gently return to your neutral position of standing upright.
- 20 repetitions a day.

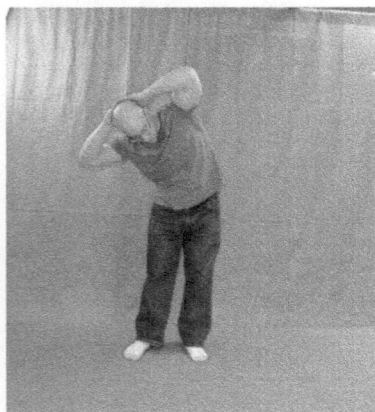

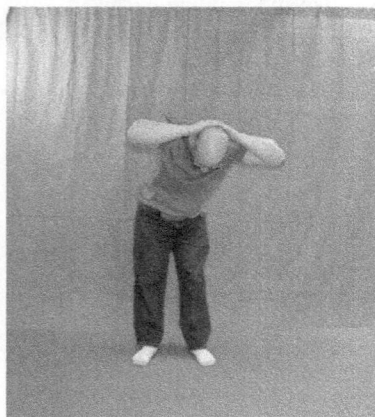

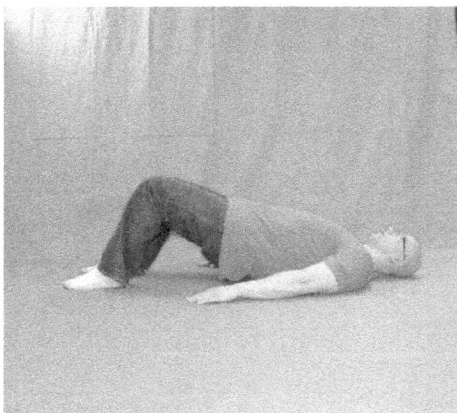

Exercise 12 (Lying Butt Lift)

- Lie down on your back.
- Gently raise your knees and pull your feet close your buttocks.
- Gently raise your pelvis as much as you can by pushing on the floor with your feet.
- Hold for 5-seconds by counting the numbers 2001 and 2002, 2003 and 2004.
- Gently lower your buttocks on the floor.
- 20 repetitions a day.

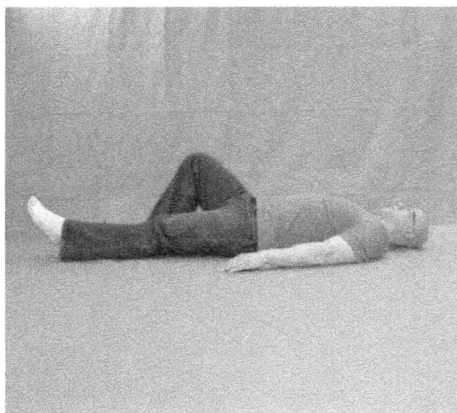

Exercise 13 (Lying Pelvis and Leg Lifts)

- Lie down on your back.
- Gently raise your right knees and pull your right foot close your buttocks.
- Gently raise your pelvis as much as you can by pushing into the floor with your right foot, while keeping your left leg in line with your torso.
- Hold for 5-seconds by counting the numbers 2001 and 2002, 2003 and 2004.
- Gently lower your buttocks and your left leg and foot back on the floor.
- Gently raise your left knee and pull your left foot close your buttocks.
- Gently raise your pelvis as much as you can by pushing on the floor with your left foot, while keeping your right leg in line with your torso.
- Hold for 5-seconds by counting the numbers 2001 and 2002, 2003 and 2004.
- Gently lower your buttocks and your right leg and foot back on the floor.
- 20 repetitions a day.

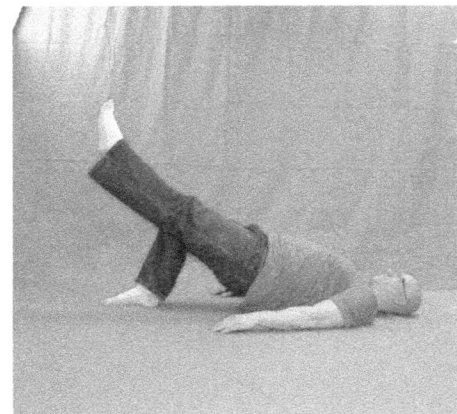

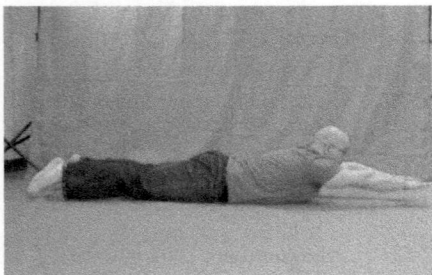

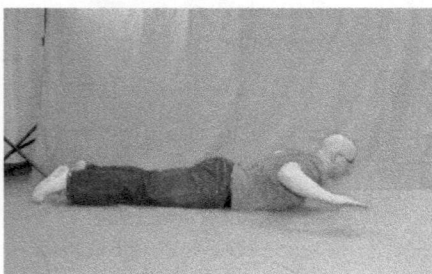

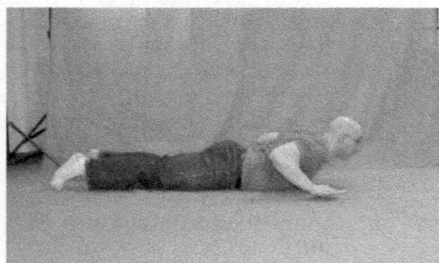

Exercise 14 (Lying Breaststrokes)

- Lie down on your stomach.
- Gently raise your head to face forward, while lifting your shoulders up and extending your arms and hands forward.
- Gently and slowly pull back your arms and hands in circular motion as if you are swimming breaststroke.
- Extend your arms and hands forward once they are back to your shoulder level.
- Repeat the circular breaststroke motions while keeping your shoulders and head up.
- 20 repetitions a day.

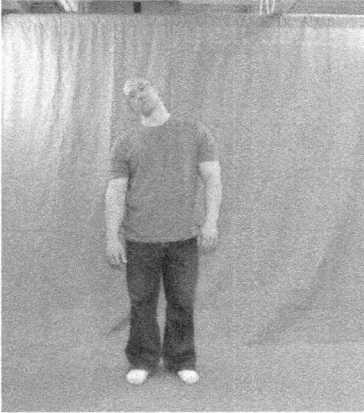

Exercise 15 (Standing Head Side to Side Tilt)
- Stand upright.
- Gently bend your head to your left, while facing forward as much as you can.
- Hold for 5-seconds by counting the numbers 2001 and 2002, 2003 and 2004.
- Gently and slowly return to neutral position.
- Repeat the same motion to your right.
- 20 repetitions a day.

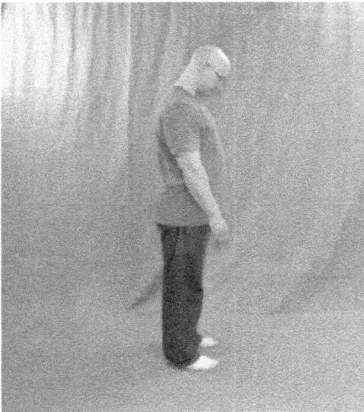

Exercise 16 (Standing Head Front to Back Tilt)
- Stand upright.
- Gently bend your head forward as much as you can.
- Hold for 5-seconds by counting the numbers 2001 and 2002, 2003 and 2004.
- Gently and slowly return to a neutral position.
- Repeat the same motion by bending your head backward.
- 20 repetitions a day.

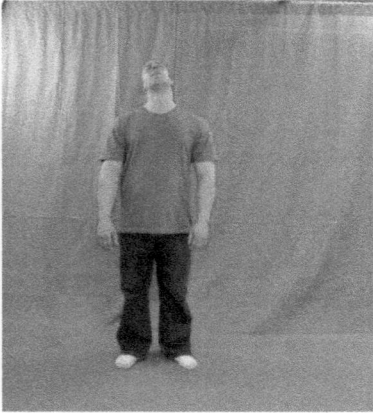

Exercise 17 (Standing Head Rotations)
- Stand upright.
- Gently rotate your head clockwise first towards your right, then your front, then your left, then your back or rear.
- Gently return to your neutral position of standing upright.
- Gently rotate your head counter-clockwise first towards your left, then your front, then your right, then your rear.
- Gently return to your neutral position of a standing upright.
- 20 repetitions a day.

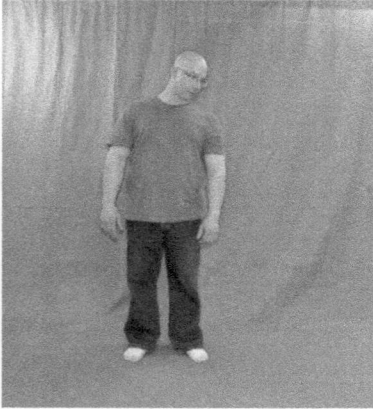

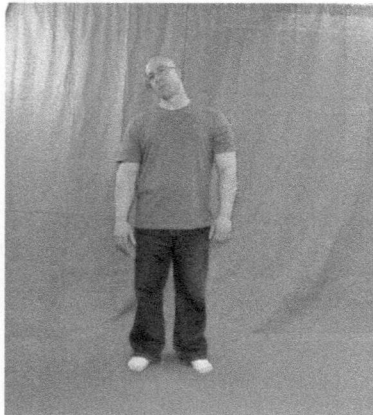

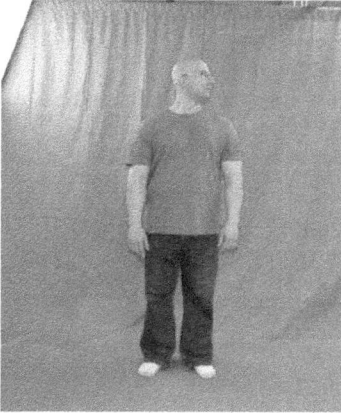

Exercise 18 (Standing Side-to-Side Head Rotation)
- Stand upright.
- Gently rotate your head to your left.
- Gently return to your neutral position of standing upright.
- Gently rotate your head to your right.
- Gently return to your neutral position of standing upright.
- 20 repetitions a day.

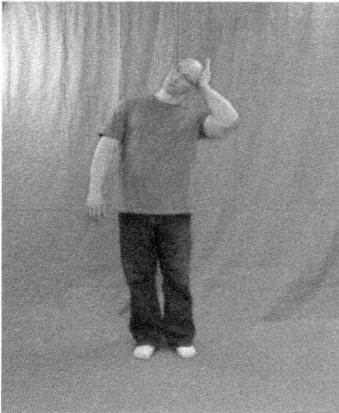

Exercise 19 (Standing Side-to-Side Head Resistance Press)
- Stand or sit upright.
- Gently press your left hand on the left head.
- Gently bend your head to your left, while applying resistance with your left hand.
- Gently return to your neutral position of standing upright.
- Gently repeat the same motion to your right with your right hand as resistance.
- 20 repetitions a day.

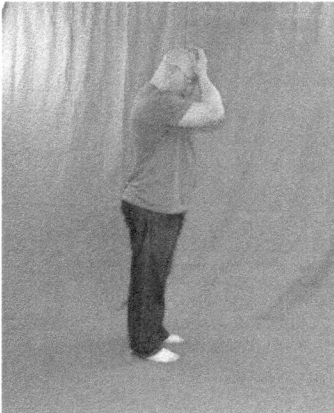

Exercise 20 (Standing Front Resistance Head Press)
- Stand or sit upright.
- Gently press you hands on your forehead.
- Gently push your head forward, while applying resistance with your hands.
- Gently return to your neutral position of standing or sitting upright.
- 20 repetitions a day.

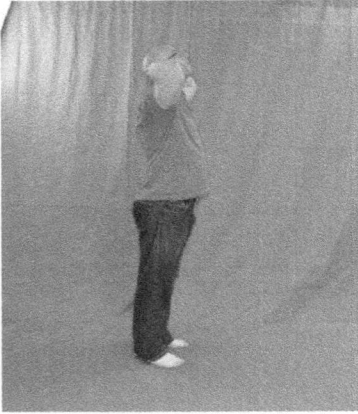

Exercise 21 (Standing Backward Resistance Head Press)

- Stand or sit upright.
- Gently press your hands on the back of your head.
- Gently push your head backward, while applying resistance with your hands.
- Gently return to your neutral position of standing or sitting upright.
- 20 repetitions a day.

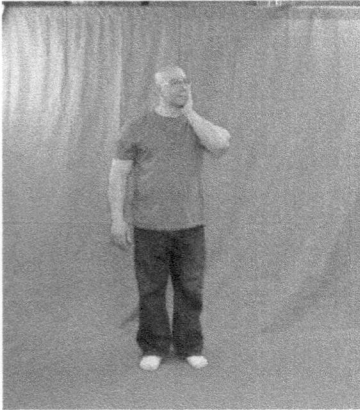

Exercise 22 (Standing Resistance Head Rotation)

- Stand or sit upright.
- Gently press your hands on your left face and jaw.
- Gently rotate your head towards your left, while applying resistance with your left hand.
- Gently return to your neutral position of standing or sitting upright.
- Gently repeat the same motion to your right with your right hand.
- 20 repetitions a day.

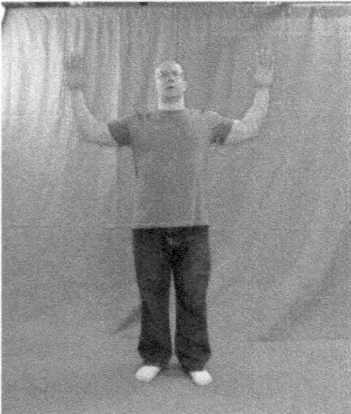

Exercise 23 (Standing Reverse Arm Stretch)

- Stand or sit upright.
- Gently raise your arms, with your upper arms being horizontal.
- Gently stretch your upper arms horizontally backward.
- Hold for 8-seconds by counting the numbers 2001 and 2002, 2003, 2004, 2005 and 2006.
- Gently return to your neutral position of standing or sitting upright, but with your arms raised.
- 20 repetitions a day.

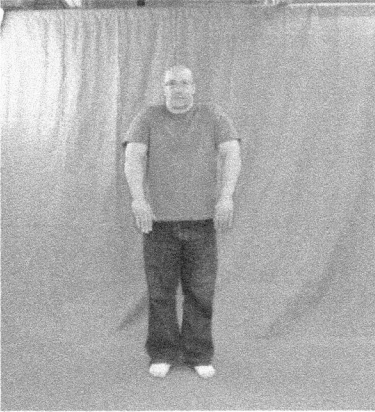

Exercise 24 (Standing Shrugs)
- Stand upright.
- Gently raise your shoulders and rotate them forward, then downward, then backward, then upward.
- Gently reverse the motion by rotating your shoulders backward, then downward, then forward, then upward.
- 20 repetitions a day.

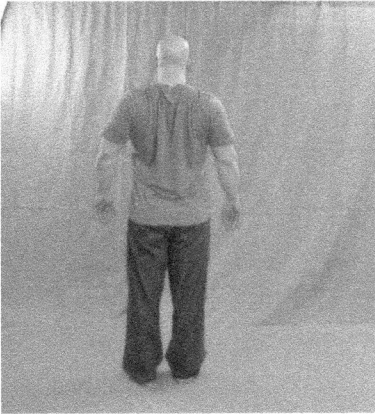

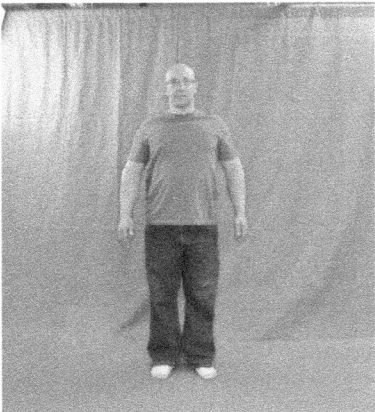

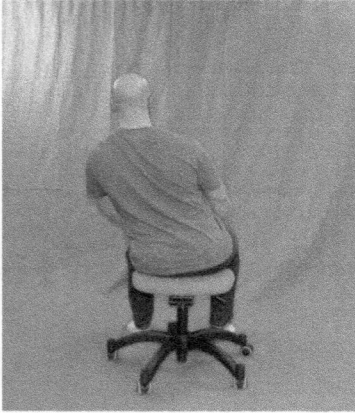

Exercise 25 (Seated Body Shifts)
- Sit upright.
- Gently shift your shoulders towards your left, while keeping your buttocks stable and your pelvis as horizontal as possible.
- Hold for 5-seconds by counting the numbers 2001 and 2002, 2003 and 2004.
- Gently and slowly return to your upright neutral position.
- Gently reverse the motion by shifting your shoulders towards your right, while keeping your buttocks stable and your pelvis as horizontal as possible.
- Hold for 5-seconds by counting the numbers 2001 and 2002, 2003 and 2004.
- Gently and slowly return to your upright neutral position.
- 20 repetitions a day.

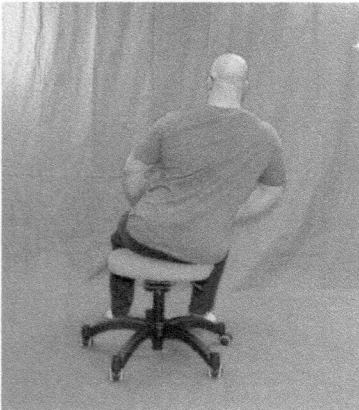

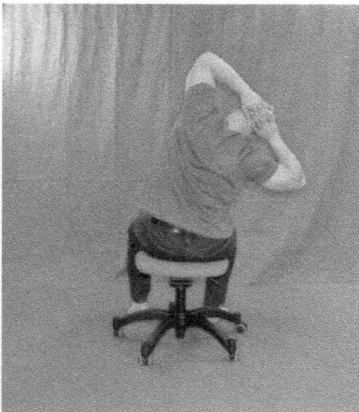

Exercise 26 (Seated Side to Side Bending)
- Sit upright.
- Bend your arms behind your head.
- Gently bend your back towards your right, while keeping your buttocks stable and your pelvis horizontal.
- Hold for 5-seconds by counting the numbers 2001 and 2002, 2003 and 2004
- Gently and slowly return to your upright neutral position.
- Gently repeat same motion by bending your back towards your left.
- 20 repetitions a day.

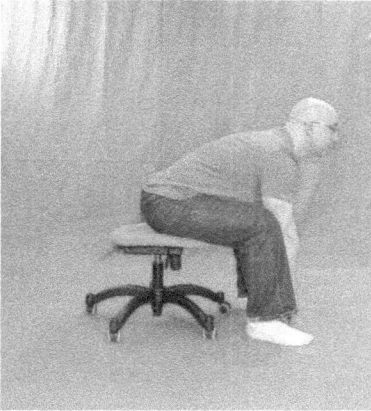

Exercise 27 (Seated Forward Hip Bending)

- Sit upright.
- Gently bend your torso forward and reach the floor with your hands, if possible.
- Hold for 5-seconds by counting the numbers 2001 and 2002, 2003 and 2004.
- Gently and slowly raise your head and let your head pull up your spine vertebra by vertebra, as if pulling up a string of beats by one of its ends.
- Hold for 5-seconds by counting the numbers 2001 and 2002, 2003 and 2004.
- 20 repetitions a day.

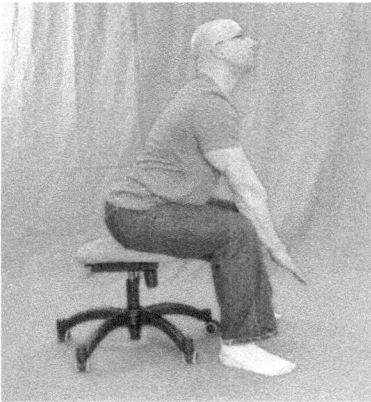

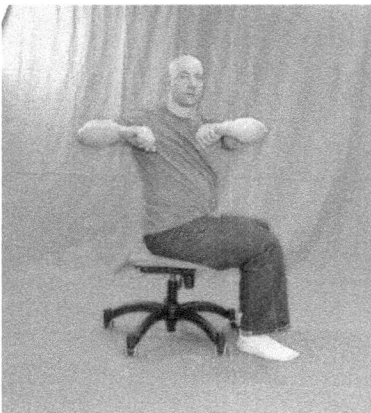

Exercise 28 (Seated Torso Twists)

- Sit upright.
- Gently twist your torso towards your right, as much as you can.
- Hold for 5-seconds by counting the numbers 2001 and 2002, 2003 and 2004.
- Gently and slowly return to your neutral position.
- Repeat the same motion by twisting your torso towards your left.
- 20 repetitions a day.

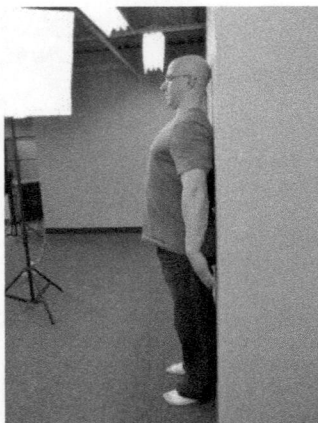

Exercise 29 (Standing Back Wall Press)

- Stand against a straight wall, while making sure that your buttocks are in touch with the wall.
- Gently move your feet backward to touch the wall.
- Gently extend your shoulder to touch the wall.
- Gently move your head backward to touch the wall, while keeping your chin back as much as you can.
- Hold for 8-seconds by counting the numbers 2001 and 2002, 2003, 2004, 2005 and 2006.
- Relax.
- 20 repetitions each day.

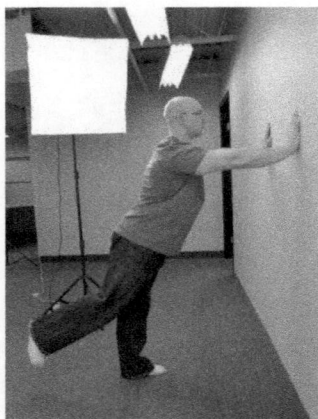

Exercise 30 (Standing Wall Backward Leg Lifts)

- Stand facing a wall at arm's length.
- Gently raise your arm to touch the wall, with your hands and slightly rest your body against the wall.
- Gently lift your right leg backward
- Hold for 8-seconds by counting the numbers 2001 and 2002, 2003, 2004, 2005 and 2006.
- Gently lower your right leg and return to a neutral position.
- Repeat the same motion with your left leg.
- 20 repetitions each day.

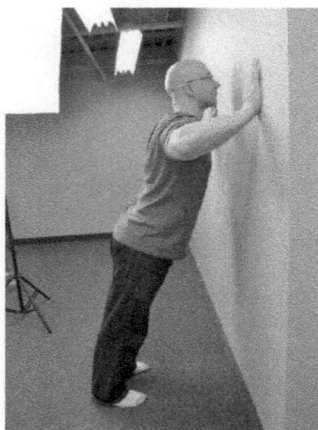

Exercise 31 (Standing Wall Push Up)

- Stand facing a wall at arm's length.
- Gently raise your arm to touch the wall, with your hands and rest your body against the wall.
- Gently bend your arms and push your chest closer to the wall.
- Hold for 8-seconds by counting the numbers 2001 and 2002, 2003, 2004, 2005 and 2006.
- Gently straighten your arms and return to neutral position.
- 20 repetitions each day.

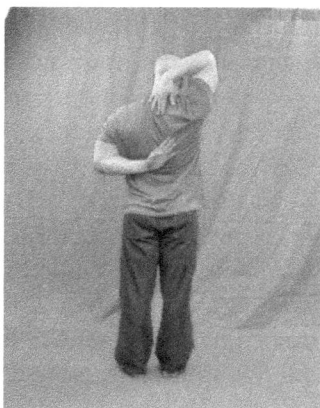

Exercise 32 (Behind the Back Arm Reach)

- Stand upright.
- Gently raise your right arm and bend it to your back over your right shoulder, while bending your left arm to your back from the left side of your lumbar area.
- Gently move your hands towards each other as much as you can.
- Hold for 8-seconds by counting the numbers 2001 and 2002, 2003, 2004, 2005 and 2006.
- Gently straighten your arms and return to a neutral position.
- Repeat the some motion with reversed arms.
- 20 repetitions each day.

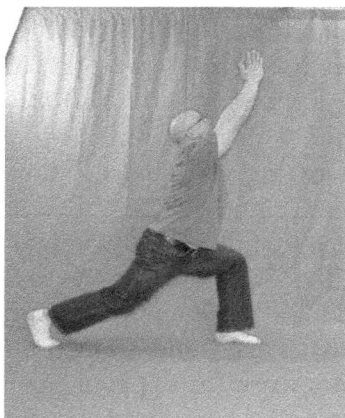

Exercise 33 (Candle Pose)

- Stand upright.
- Gently take a large step forward, with your left foot and lower your body.
- Gently extend your arms forward and upward with your hands touching each other and pointing to the mid day sun, as if there is an invisible string between your fingers and the sun pulling your body upward.
- Hold for 8-seconds by counting the numbers 2001 and 2002, 2003, 2004, 2005 and 2006.
- Gently return to a neutral position.
- 20 repetitions each day.

2. Pilates Exercises

Pilates is a concept and method of physical exercises created by German gymnast, author, and inventor Joseph Pilates. It is said that because of the effectiveness of his fitness concept and method, most of his fellow mates who learned and practiced his exercises were in such good physical health that they survived the 1918 flu pandemic.

Many back pain sufferers have found Pilates exercises highly effective to help contain their pain. According to Beth Glosten, MD, patients with pain due to excessive movement, spinal degeneration, and postural asymmetry are most likely to benefit from a Pilates exercise program.

After all, Pilates focuses on improving your spinal alignment and strengthening your core. A poor alignment of the spine and a weak core are the causes for many back pains.

Pilates helps you improve your body's flexibility, muscle strength, endurance, and the stability of your back and your core muscles, hips, legs, arms, and abdominals. It emphasizes spinal and pelvic alignment, proper breathing, good coordination, and balance.

A study published in the 2014 *European Journal of Physical and Rehabilitation Medicine* has: "found an important improvement of pain, disability, and physical and psychological perception of health in individuals who did the daily sessions of Pilates."

"This study suggests that a daily Pilates program is effective for the management of CLBP (chronic lower back pain). On the other hand, the inactivity contributes to further worsening, inducing a vicious cycle, in which pain and physical activity intolerance follow each other."

You may also come across studies arguing that the effectiveness of Pilates is still inconclusive. The reality is that the human body is a complex organic structure. Some individuals respond to certain approaches while others don't. The fact that Pilates and other non-chemical and non-surgical approaches do not work for all people may be a good thing for back pain sufferers, because such approaches do not touch upon the most fundamental biological building blocks of our bodies, such as using a chemical to numb a nerve, or using a scalpel to take out a smashed vertebra.

Drugs and spinal implants as a "source of a cure" can be standardized, by type of chemical, its dosage, its formulation, or its type of element and strength. A non-drug and non-surgical care solution, as a "source of a cure" can hardly be standardized, as a practitioner's knowledge level, skill level, and experience level can be quantified.

The point here is that Pilates does work for many people as indicated by many studies. Back pain sufferers simply need to learn and explore the possibilities to see if it would work for them, instead of being told that you have to live with your pain for the rest of your life.

Anyone can practice and benefit from Pilates exercises, whether you are physically weak or super strong. Whether you are novice or a master. And whether you have or do not have back pain. Find a good Pilates teacher and try the exercises out. Only actual trials can tell you whether or not or how much you can benefit for this approach.

3. Alexander Technique

The Alexander Technique was originated by Australian singer, Frederick Matthias Alexander, towards the end of the 19th century.

The Alexander Technique combines lessons and exercises to help people better use their muscles, better conduct daily activities, improve their physical habits, improve proprioceptive awareness, and to better sense the warning signals of bodily tension and stress.

The Alexander Technique lessons offer individualized training to develop lifelong skills for self-care, by helping people recognize, understand, and avoid poor habits affecting posture and neuromuscular coordination. Lessons involve personalized assessment and improvement of habitual musculoskeletal use, with a special focus on releasing unwanted head, neck, and spinal muscle tension.

A *British Medical Journal* study in 2008, took 579 patients with chronic or recurrent lower back pain and showed that the Alexander Technique lessons helped patients effectively reduce lower back pain and significantly improved their quality of life, with long-lasting effects. It showed after six lessons in of the Alexander Technique, patients retained its effectiveness for one-year. While six sessions of massage were much less effective one-year later.

The long-term benefits of the Alexander Technique are not surprising because it focuses on resolving the causes of many back pains by teaching patients how to better use their bodies, improve their bodies' biomechanics, and be better in tuned with their bodies.

A study published in the 2012 *International Journal of Clinical Practice* by Woodman and Moore, also showed that: "strong evidence exists for the effectiveness of [the] Alexander Technique lessons for chronic back pain."

4. Feldenkrais Method

The Feldenkrais Method was originated by Moshé Feldenkrais (1904 to 1984). Like the Alexander Technique, Feldenkrais is an educational system for encouraging the right movements of the human body.

Feldenkrais helps students reduce pain or limitations in movement, improve physical function, and promote general wellbeing, by increasing their kinesthetic and proprioceptive self-awareness of functional movement.

A 1992 study regarding the Feldenkrais Method and back pain, by author Bernard Lake, found that after four Feldenkrais sessions, 76 percent of participants with chronic lower back pain had improved sufficiently to conduct normal daily activities.

A study published in a 2011 issue of *Journal Bodywork Movement Therapies*, found the Feldenkrais Method helped improve students' ability to perform everyday tasks, reduce levels of pain and improve their quality of life.

5. Tai Chi

Tai Chi is an ancient form of fitness exercises, mental focus and martial arts. It is an ideal form of exercise for relieving and preventing back pain. It is gentle, slow moving, fluid, and comprehensive. Tai Chi emphasizes a stable stance for the back, the pelvis and the legs. It is very helpful in helping develop good posture, strengthening the deep stabilizing muscles in the back, and enhancing the flexibility of the back.

Tai Chi contributes to chronic pain management in several major areas: adaptive exercise, postural improvement, back strength and core stability enhancement, and mind-body interaction.

A study published in 2011 in *Arthritis Care & Research*, found that: "a 10-week Tai Chi program improved pain and disability outcomes and can be considered a safe and effective intervention for those experiencing long-term lower back pain symptoms." Study reviews also reveal that Tai Chi may be effective in the battle against osteoarthritis and fibromyalgia.

There are five main styles of Tai Chi. Some are more health oriented, while others are combat or competition oriented. For relief and prevention of back pain, you may wish to choose a style that is more oriented towards health and fitness.

Yang Style Tai Chi was created by Yang Lu-ch'an (1799 to 1872). Due to the influence and success of Yang Luchan and Yang Tai Chi, three other main styles of Tai Chi except Chen Tai Chi, claim to originate from Yang Tai Chi. It is the most widely practiced form of Tai Chi worldwide. It is open, gentle, fluid, and even paced. It is particularly suited to help enhance health, posture, and stamina.

Wu Tai Chi was founded by Wu Ch'uan-yu (1834 to1902), and is more sophisticated and has a stronger mental exercise component. It is the second most widely practiced Tai Chi style. It is practiced for both its health and its mental enhancement benefits.

Chen Style Tai Chi is the oldest style created by Chen Wangting (1580 to 1660). While Chen is the original style of Tai Chi, it is today ranked as the third most popular style of Tai Chi. It has the strongest martial art roots and combative components than any other style of Tai Chi. It combines the soft and slow, with the hard and fast. It is the best for those who want something exciting. If you do choose to learn the Chen Tai Chi Style, try to do the soft and slow exercises at first. Once you are confident that your back can take it, you may move to practice the hard and fast and the combative components of this style.

As the author of this book, I am a personal fan of this style of Tai Chi, and have a wonderful teacher Master Yan, PhD, in Markham, Ontario, Canada. Dr. Yan (with a Tai Chi name Master Chen given by his Grand Master) is a 12th generation Chen's Tai Chi inheritor – one of the eighteen inheritor disciples of Grand Master Chen Zhenglei. One of his teachings that may be most beneficial to back pain sufferers or preventers is to disengage the force applied upon your body that is to reduce the resistance of your body to the foreign force, as much and as quickly as possible.

Sun Tai Chi was founded by Sun Lu-t'ang (1861 to 1932). Sun style is the fourth most practiced style of Tai Chi. It is agile with a higher stance and large foot work. It may be easier for beginners. It is often considered as being more suitable for health enhancement and rehabilitation.

Wu-Hao Style Tai Chi was founded by Wu Yu-hsiang (1813 to

1880) who was a student of Yang Tai Chi. Wu-Hao Tai Chi is the least practiced major style of Tai Chi.

Visit some masters or teachers of various styles of Tai Chi and do some sample practices to find the style that suits you the most. If your main aim is to relieve back pain, your best initial bet may be Yang Style Tai Chi, Wu Style Tai Chi, or Sun Style Tai Chi.

6. Yoga

Yoga is an ancient form of health preservation that predates Tai Chi. It may have emerged as early as 500 to 200 BCE. It focuses on physical, mental, and spiritual enhancement. But its ultimate goal is spiritual in nature – liberation.

A study of adults with chronic lower back pain that was published by the Boston University Medical Center in 2009, found: "pain scores for the yoga participants decreased by one-third compared to the control group, which decreased by only five percent. Whereas pain medication use in the control group did not change, yoga participants' use of pain medicines decreased by 80 percent. Improvement in function was also greater for yoga participants but was not statistically significant."

A study published by the University of Duisburg-Essen, Essen, Germany, in 2013 had: "found strong evidence for short-term effectiveness and moderate evidence for long-term effectiveness of yoga for chronic lower back pain in the most important patient-centered outcomes. Yoga can be recommended as an additional therapy to chronic lower back pain patients."

A study published in *Evidence Based Complement Alternative Medicine* in 2013, found interestingly that 12-weeks of once-weekly yoga classes were similarly effective as twice-weekly classes. It seems to indicate that the most important thing with Yoga is just to do it. Whether once or twice a week is not important.

There are many different types of Yoga, from gentle and slow to rigorous and challenging. Each style has a large number of levels of difficulties. Because of the wide ranging style, highly different approaches, and high number of levels of difficulty in each style, back pain sufferers must be careful in selecting the right type and level to practice.

You want to begin with a type of yoga that incorporates some gentle and slow movements, but is gentle on the back. And you want to begin at an entry level and gradually build up your physique and skills. It may be better for you to find a class that is specially designed for back pain sufferers. If you don't love a style of yoga after your first class, try other teachers, as one teacher's class, even of the same type, can vary significantly from the next.

It will be greatly helpful to yourself and the teacher to tell her or him about your back condition to allow the teacher to tailor your exercises to your specific condition. Always make sure that you are not making your back too sore. While no pain, no gain may be true, excessive pain should be avoided. You must find a balance between movement and pain.

Types of Yoga

Aerial: a hammock based yoga practice. Fun but some of its movements may not be suitable for back pain sufferers.

Anusara: is based on slow movements and stretches. Many of its exercises are highly beneficial to strengthen the back and prevent back pain, however, some of the exercises may be too strenuous to back pain sufferers.

Ashtanga: this type of yoga is highly vigorous. It is good for back pain prevention. Back pain sufferers should be careful about practicing it.

Bikram: a modern version of hot yoga that practices various poses in heated studios. Most of the poses should be helpful to the back. However, back pain sufferers need to try to do poses in short durations. Keep transitioning from one pose to another gently, and slowly, but continuously.

Hatha: is the foundation for many yoga styles. It incorporates slow movements and stretches. Good for beginners. Make sure you keep moving, and do not hold on to one position for too long. Initially 5-seconds should be your maximum. This maximum can be extended as you progress in your training over a period of weeks or months.

Hot Yoga: is done in a heated environment of 80 to 105 degree Fahrenheit studios with durations lasting 60 to 90 minutes. Your body will be more relaxed because of the heat. Many practitioners find hot yoga particularly effective in pain relief.

Iyengar: is a modern version of Hatha Yoga with systemized poses and difficulty levels. Specially designed for many people to learn Yoga.

Kundalini: Kundalini means "a spiritual energy or life force located at the base of the spine." It is a gentle form of yoga, focusing on meditation and breathing accompanied with gentle and slow back strengthening and back revitalizing movements.

Vinyasa flow: Vinyasa movements flow smoothly and are almost dance-like.

Yin: Yin yoga is the yoga of stretches. It aims for deep stretches and tends to hold on a stretched pose for a longer time to improve flexibility. Most of the stretches are focused on the hip and the back.

If you have pain relief as your main purpose of practicing yoga, you may want to first try hot yoga, hatha yoga, Kundalini yoga, and Iyengar yoga. Make sure you find a qualified teacher, who is experienced with teaching students with back pain. It is even better if you can find a teacher who has had successful experiences in teaching students with similar kinds of back conditions to yours.

7. Swimming
Swimming is one the best and safest exercises to relieve or prevent back pain.

Virtually anything you do in the water, except prolonged breaststrokes, will be good for your back. Just make sure that you don't slip and fall on a wet floor.

Water allows your body to relax. Water offers your body a soothing massage.

8. Gentle Dancing
One of the best activities is to dance, uncompetitive, gentle dance or ball room dance. Competitive dance is prone to back injuries and pain due to extreme twisting, flexion and extension of the back, and stressful jumping, diving and lifting actions.

Gentle ball room dancing helps you strengthen your back and your core. It also helps you to:

- Improve the flexibility of your spine,
- Keep your discs hydrated,
- Slow down the aging process of your spine,
- Stay in a good mood and reduce and prevent depression,
- Maintain your equilibrium or functional balance,
- Reduce and prevent slipping and falling.

Best of all you are playing and having fun. You won't even notice your effort in improving your back. Time will pass in a blink of an eye. You can dance almost anywhere you like, with or without a partner. You don't have to do it precisely right. Start dancing today. You can do it. Turn on the music now. And start dancing. Just do it, today. You can always debate me or thank me later.

PART FOUR
YOU ARE YOUR SPINE

Read this chapter, if you ever wonder why you should take care of your back, or if you still have any doubt about the importance of taking care of your back and spine.

1

Your Spine Is Your Freedom

The fact is that you can function reasonably well, live relatively independently, even become an inspirational hero, if you lose your teeth, ears, eyes, or a hand, arm, foot, leg, even all of your limbs.

The great inspirational speaker Nick Vujicic is an excellent example. Despite being born with no arms and virtually no legs, he has persevered. He not only leads a happy and productive life, but also inspires millions from around the world to persevere and fight any handicaps handed to them in life.

However, if you lose your spine, your internal organs will be dropped on top of each other like a pile of dirty laundry, and you would literally become a meat ball. Furthermore, the protection of your spinal cord will be lost. Your spinal cord and the nerves will be damaged and destroyed and none of your vital organs will work.

It's hard to imagine how anyone could function without a spine, even a great hero, such as Nick: "The famous Professor Stephen Hawking is a leading astro-physicist and inspirational figure despite his spinal issues," you may say. However, even Professor Hawkings' spine still has a certain degree of function. Imagine how much more he could have achieved, if he had a better spine.

"You are your spine," is no cliché. And it is critical to remember that, if you don't take care of your back, you will outlive your spine.

A healthy spine allows you mobility and the ability to do the things you want to, even including taking care of yourself. Spinal issues range greatly from improper alignment to degenerative spinal discs, to spinal cord injury. Any issue with your spine may severely limit your freedom. Improper alignment of your spine may lead to interference of your nerves, which can result in a variety of health issues, such as back pain, sciatic pain, numb hands, malfunction of your organs, and paralyzed extremities.

Once your spinal health is in question, you may have difficulties lifting your arms to feed yourself, you may not even be able to grab and hold your toothbrush. Your back pain may make it difficult to walk your dog, to visit your favorite shops, or to exercise at your favorite gym. You may have difficulty sitting comfortably at your dinner table to enjoy your meals, sitting on your couch to watch your favorite TV shows, taking a ride in your car to visit your family or friends, or boarding an airplane for a vacation. Of course, for those whose spinal cord is injured, it may be even more difficult to sit up independently.

Spinal issues not only limit the patients in their physical freedom, but also limit their social freedom. Back pain sufferers often feel socially isolated. They are not able meet their friends as often as they would like. They are limited in joining their friends for activities, such as going for a walk in the park.

Back pain doesn't discriminate. Anyone can be affected by it, whether you have good genes or not, whether you are young or not, whether you are wealthy or not, whether you're male or female, whether you are born fit or not, whether you have a naturally good physique or not, whether you are especially good looking or not, whether you have a PhD degree or not, whether you are famous or not.

2

Your Spine Is Your Sexuality

It is not that you can't explore your sexuality with your partner to the fullest, or simply have a few less sex sessions per month, without a good spine. It is that your drive and joy of sexuality is killed. If you are a young or middle-aged person, poor sexual drive and loss of joy of sexuality will put stress on your relationship that nothing else can compensate, and will put a dent in your self-confidence and expression that no other means could balance.

Studies have shown that sexuality is profoundly disturbed in chronic low back pain patients and that both their sexual intercourse and sexual quality of life were affected.

Negatively affected sexuality also tends to contribute to depression, which in turn puts stress on relationships, work productivity, and team collaboration.

People tend to be silent about a troubled sex life due to back pain. However, such silence further exaggerates the problem itself. Talk to your partner about the situation openly, if your sex life is affected by back pain. Let your partner know your limitations. Try different positions and places that would be easier for you. Prepare your body physically. Plan with your partner. Soothe your back in advance. Take your time. Take advantage of sex toys and aids. Don't stress yourself too much. Know when to say no, and know when to stop. You are in a relationship for a longer-term. Think about the sustainability of your sex life.

3

Your Spine Is Your Vitality

Needless to say, back pain quickly and negatively affects the essential ingredients of your vitality and happiness. Studies have found that it has an immediate impact on your:

- Mood
- Spirit
- Vigor
- Personal energy
- Physical stamina
- Physical mobility
- Initiative
- Joy
- Laughter
- Liveliness
- Sexuality
- Self confidence
- Self-expression

Besides the brain and heart, one could hardly find any other body part that can have such a profound, varied and far reaching impacts, when troubled. However, in the case of the spine, even relatively mild trouble, such as a herniated disc can have such effects.

Your spine is not only vulnerable, but literally critical to your vitality and happiness.

4

Your Spine Is Your Financial Wealth

Someone may say "I have a healthy spine, but I don't have much money. How could you say my spine is my wealth?" You can rest assured that if you do have a poor spine or back pain, you will have a lot less money at your disposal, or a lot more debt. Your back pain will either eat you alive financially, emotionally, or both.

Spine disorders and back pain are highly pervasive. It is the leading cause for visiting a doctor's office, second only to cough and flu. Thirty percent of all American adults are afflicted by them each year. Eighty percent of all people will have an acute episode of back pain in their lifetime. The irony is that most back pain can be traced back to non-serious causes. Most of them are mechanical in nature. And most of them can be prevented and avoided by simple awareness and preventative measures.

It is also highly costly. According to the American Academy of Orthopedic Surgeons, American back pain sufferers spend a staggering $200USD Billion on directly treating back pain, which means that it costs a person afflicted with back pain an average of $2,890USD to treat their back pain each year. Patients who suffer from bad backs are hit harder. They spend an average of $6,096USD in 2005, an increase of 65 percent from $4,795USD in 1997 (after being adjusted for inflation) according to the 2011 *Annals of Internal Medicine* by the American College of Physicians.

Despite the increased costs, adults with spine pain reported no improvement and in some cases even worse scores when evaluated for mental health, physical functioning, work or school limitations and social limitations from 1997 to 2005, according to the above paper.

The 2013 back pain survey of 14,000 people who had at least one episode of back pain in the previous 12-months found while most of the survey's participants had severely limiting pain for less than a week, 35 percent of them never consulted a professional.

The report also found that many of those with more prolonged pain who didn't see a health-care professional said it was because of cost concerns.

Imagine how much more you could do with an extra $6,000 after tax money in your pocket. A nice vacation? Pay off debt? Better nutrition? Nicer apartment? More time with family? And much more.

If the above statistics are not enough, consider this: back pain is one of the leading reasons for single cause disability. How would your financial health look if you were prematurely disabled?

5

Your Spine Is Your Career

While one will be greatly limited in what she/he could do professionally when severe spinal disorder strikes, spinal disorders also greatly affect productivity. Back pain and injury are the biggest causes for missed work days in America. Studies indicate that 1 out every 10 work days missed in America is due to back pain. Often even minor spinal disorders can significantly impact productivity. Back aches and pains often distract the sufferers from work and tasks at hand, limit the range of physical tasks they can perform, limit the physical destinations they can reach, and limit the level of productivity they can achieve, whether in one's professional or personal lives.

A healthy spine is indeed an essential condition for your professional and personal productivity. Of course, there are exceptions, such as Sam Sullivan, the former mayor of Vancouver, BC, Canada, who sustained a neck injury while skiing and has been severely paralyzed from the neck down since age 19. Although permanently bound to his wheelchair, he sat up six non-profit organizations dedicated to improving the quality of life for disabled people in North America, before becoming the mayor of Vancouver.

But even for Sam Sullivan, his professional and personal freedom and success would be completely different, had he not been physically limited by his spinal issues.

If you have never had a back problem, you may say: "Spinal cord issues are rare and will not happen to me. Back pain won't have that kind of impact on my life, and doesn't scare me." Don't be so fast to draw this conclusion.

Severe or chronic back pains often greatly compromise our ability to reach our full potential. It greatly affects our ability and availability to work. It greatly affects our concentration in whatever we do. It greatly limits our choice of things that we could possibly engage in. It greatly affects our relationships. It greatly affects our moods, emotions, self-confidence, and happiness.

A study published in JAMA (*The Journal of the American Medical Association*) in 2003, shows that back pain sufferers lost an average of 5.2 hours of productive time per week. Total lost productive time from back pain among active workers costs an estimated $17.9 Billion each year in America alone. In 2010, this equivalent cost had increased to $27 Billion. Among the 155 million total US workforce, an astonishing 1.34 billion productive hours are lost due to back pain each year. The lost work hours due to missed work days counts an additional 101.8 million workdays and 814.4 million hours owing to back pain each year in the US.

6

Your Spine Is Your Life Insurance

Spinal issues often affect quality of life far more than what one may normally realize. Aside from the effects of limited range of physical and social freedom, of compromised sleep and rest in the night, of reduced levels of productivity, of level of wellbeing, even independent living, chronic back pain may also result in compromised appetite, reduced satisfaction with food intake, and ironically also obesity.

According to Dr. Shane Burch, an assistant professor at University of California San Francisco department of orthopaedic surgery, severe on-going back pain may put your level of physical capacity and quality of life below that of seniors 75-years or older, who are not afflicted by any back pain or serious medical conditions. A study shows that the utility score, which reflects the level of your body's physical capability to function in daily life, of patients with severe back pain is around an average of 0.5 (with 0.0 as the score for dead people, and 1.0 is the score assigned to people with perfect health). While healthy seniors of 75-years plus have an average score of 0.65, (about 30 percent higher than the people with back pain.) Literally, severe back pain can turn you into an old man or old lady overnight, as far as the level of utility of your body is concerned.

Studies have shown that people with chronic lower back pain often have changes in the areas of the brain that are associated with food and pleasure. Dr. Paul Geha, lead author of a new clinical study at the Yale University School of Medicine in New Haven, Connecticut, said people with chronic back pain might not be able to derive as much pleasure from eating as others.

"Patients who suffer from chronic lower back pain might be at risk of overeating, especially from the highly palatable, energy dense food," Dr. Geha told Reuters Health.

"This study, however, proposes the argument that chronic lower back pain affects a patient's relationship with food such that the patient's pleasure from eating is decreased and the patient's ability to know when to stop eating is also decreased, thereby leading to overeating and weight gain," affirmed Dr. Naum Shaparin, director of Pain Service at Montefiore Medical Center in Bronx, New York in a conversation with Reuter Health.

Chronic lower back pain is very common in the United States. According to the American Academy of Orthopedic Surgeons (AAOS), 30 percent of American adults are afflicted by lower back pain annually, and back pain is the leading cause for visits to doctors, second only to cold and flu. Chances are that one in every three adult friends you know is afflicted with back pain.

"Lower back pain, in general, is one of the most common reasons for a doctor's visit, both in the office and the emergency department," confirmed Dr. Naum Shaparin.

Some studies even show that about a quarter of adults report experiencing back pain for one day in the last three months, indicated Dr. Amir Qaseem, MD, PhD, director of clinical policy with the American College of Physicians' medical education division.

In a 2013 survey of over 14,000 people that had suffered lower back pain, in the previous 12 months that never had back surgery, the Consumer Reports Health Ratings Center found that more than half said the pain severely limited their daily routine for a week or longer, and 88 percent said it recurred throughout the year. The survey also found that 46 percent of back pain sufferers said that back pain interfered with their sleep, 31 percent reported that it thwarted their efforts to maintain a healthy weight, and 24 percent said that it hampered their sex life.

A study published in *Spinal Cord* in 2013, found that the majority of both male and female chronic lower back pain patients experienced sexual problems, which is considerably higher than the rates among the healthy population. The study involved 702 patients with chronic lower back pain and 888 healthy individuals and showed that the prevalence of sexual problems in female patients with chronic lower back pain was twice as high as the corresponding figure for healthy women (71.1 percent versus 36.8 percent), and that erectile dysfunction among male patients with chronic lower back pain was more than twice as frequent when compared to healthy men (59.5 percent versus 24.5 percent).

Back pain does not only directly cause sexual problems, but also indirectly causes sexual problems among back pain patients through the pain management drugs taken by the patients, such as opioid painkillers and the side effects of back pain, such as depressive disorder.

A study published in a 2013 *British Medical Journal*: "found that the probability of receiving drugs for erectile dysfunction or testosterone replacement increased with increased dose and duration of opioid treatment." The researchers: "estimated that long-term use of opioid painkillers was linked to a 45 percent increase in the chance of erection problems. Patients prescribed the highest doses of opioids (≥120 mg of morphine equivalents per day) were 58 percent more likely to have drug treatment for erectile dysfunction or low testosterone. Depressive disorders and the use of sedatives or hypnotics were also associated with prescriptions for erectile dysfunction or reduced replacement."

Taking good care of your spine will help reduce visits to doctors' offices, help you do more of what you want, help you enjoy more of what you do, and help you achieve more in what you do.

Back pain and spinal problems have far more consequences than the examples mentioned above. The incomplete list below provides a little taste of the wide range of the consequences:

- Disturbance of sleep quality,
- Sitting comfort,
- Sleeping comfort – poor rejuvenation, recovery,
- Deconditioning of the body,
- Disability,
- Restricted range of motion,

- Restricted daily activity,
- Restricted recreation,
- Restricted travel,
- Restricted relationship building and sexuality,
- Restricted neuromuscular stimulation and exercises – a functional decline,
- Restricted self-care,
- Restricted care of family,
- Restricted work adaptability, if not disabled,
- Restricted job opportunity,
- Affects one's emotion, and
- Affects one's social functioning.

7

No One Is Above The Spine

Everyone this is subject to spinal failure, no matter how famous you are, how much money you have, or how strong your body is. Spinal problems can lead to devastating consequences no matter who you are. No one is above the spine. No one could have any inherent immunity against spinal problems, if he or she takes the spine for granted.

Many famous and well-off celebrities suffered from spinal injuries and back pain.

Neymar

In the critical soccer World Cup match between Brazil and Columbia, Brazil's best scorer, Neymar da Silva Santos Júnior was injured with a fractured vertebra in his back. Deeply entrenched in excruciating pain, he was taken off the field. At the next match against Germany, the Brazilian team swore to fight for Neymar and the Brazilian fans wore Neymar face masks to show the world, that Germany was up against a nation of "Neynars," and that Brazil will win.

Unfortunately, Brazil not only lost the game but also suffered a historical and humiliating score of 1-7. As a result, the Brazilian team lost their hope of winning the world cup on their home soil -- a terrible nightmare for at least half of a century until the next opportunity came along.

Back injury not only cost Neymar the opportunity to continue his performance in the World Cup, it crushed Brazil's national dream of winning the Cup on its home soil and led to a national tragedy. The entire nation was in tears for the dashed hope.

In this case, not only the interest of Neymar was affected, but the interest of an entire nation and the hearts of 300 million people were on the line.

Back injuries not only affect those people with a weak back, but also people with arguably the strongest back in the world.

Christopher Reeve

One of the most famous persons disabled by spinal problems in recent time was Superman movie star, Christopher D'Olier Reeve. He was an American actor, film director, producer, screenwriter, author and activist.

His spinal cord was injured during an equestrian competition in Virginia on May 27, 1995. He was bound to a wheelchair and breathing apparatus for the rest of his life. However, his quadriplegia didn't stop him. He worked tirelessly, championing the cause of people with spinal cord injuries, and fighting for human embryonic stem cell research. He founded the Christopher Reeve Foundation and co-founded the Reeve-Irvine Research Center.

Evgeni Plushenko

A hero to Russia, figure skater Evegeni Plushenko won the Olympic Gold medal in 2006 and the silver medals in both 2002 and 2010. He was forced out of the men's short program at the 2014 Sochi Olympic games because of back pain.

Plushenko who was only 31, told reporters that he was in too much pain to take part in the men's competition.

"I need a big rest now, and to have some treatment," he said. "Then I need to start my rehabilitation. I have already had four pills today." At the time, pain stricken, Plyshenko indicated that his Olympic career was probably over, due to back pain.

How sad, if you don't take care of your back, it will not take care of you when you need it. This even happens with the best of the top

Olympians. Take care of your back before it lets you down, even if you think that you are as strong as Plushenko.

Henrik Zetterberg

A hero to Detroit Red Wings hockey fans, and the captain of the famed hockey team, Henrik Zetterberg was forced to withdraw from the Sochi 2014 Olympics Games because of back pain. He said his back pain suddenly became "20 times worse" than what he experienced before. He has been plagued by back pain due to a herniated disc for years. But the final straw may have ended the United States hope for the gold medal in the men's hockey in Sochi.

"I felt it a bit after the game against the Czech Republic, but no more than usual," Zetterberg told Swedish newspaper *Aftonbladet*. "But on Thursday, it got worse and worse and now it is 20 times worse than before. ... It hurts at the slightest movement. Really disappointing."

Back pain requires and deserves immediate attention. Putting up with it or forcing the body into intense physical activities, may result in devastating consequences. Take it easy and pay attention to your back immediately, even if you can put up with it. Don't take chances, if you are not in a life or death situation.

Paula Abdul

A former judge on the TV show *American Idol* and a famous singer, dancer and, choreographer, Paula Abdul has suffered from severe chronic pain for over two decades. Her condition was caused by a cheerleading injury in high school. It was further aggravated by her involvement in a number of car accidents. Abdul was eventually diagnosed with a condition known as Complex Regional Pain Syndrome.

Melanie Griffith

The Oscar-nominated actress was involved in a car accident in her twenties, which left her with chronic neck and back pain. The lingering pain has caused her to get addicted to pain relief medications, further complicating her condition.

Brett Favre

A renowned football player and a three-time NFL MVP winner,

Favre was plagued by chronic pain caused by bone spurs on his ankle. He underwent surgery twice, in addition to other measures, to cope with his condition.

Jerry Lewis
A comedy legend, Jerry Lewis suffered from chronic back pain for over 30-years. His condition was further complicated when he damaged his spine during a comedy routine in 1965.

Anna Nicole Smith
The deceased actress and model reportedly suffered from chronic pain for a significant part of her life. In the process of coping with her pain, she became addicted to pain relief medications and other drugs.

Jennifer Lopez
American actress and singer, "J. Lo" was treated for back pain while in Argentina for part of her "Dance Again" Tour.

Bo Derek
The drop-dead gorgeous blonde played the perfect woman in the 1979 movie *10*, but off-screen, pain made Bo Derek's life far from ideal. A herniated disc from years of horseback riding caused chronic lower back pain. In 2003, she was featured in a photo exhibit of celebrities living with pain. The "Many Faces of Pain" exhibit toured the country, raising awareness about proper pain management.

Bono
The front man of the Irish rock band, U2, suffered debilitating back pain in 2010 while rehearsing for an upcoming tour. Bono had emergency back surgery because of severe compression of the sciatic nerve, an injury that caused sudden partial paralysis, according to doctors. After weeks of pain management and rehabilitation, U2 and Bono were able to resume their world-wide concert tour.

George Clooney
The famous actor suffered a debilitating back injury, while filming the 2005 thriller *Syriana*. Hitting his head on the floor during an intensely violent scene, he tore the dura -- the wrap around the spine that

holds in spinal fluids -- and told reporters that, prior to a number of corrective surgeries, the pain was so bad that he thought: "ending it all" seemed like a viable option. Despite undergoing surgery and reinforcing his spine with bolts, Clooney says the injury has never completely healed, forcing the 50-year-old star to drop out of filmmaker Steven Soderbergh's version of the 1960s spy series *The Man from U.N.C.L.E.*

According to Eonline.com, "He said he just can't do the action and stunt scenes," revealed an U.N.C.L.E. source who's familiar with the actor's health condition. "In fact, I think he's planning on having another operation during the time he would have been filming."

Jennifer Grey

The 2010 *Dancing with the Stars* champ suffered chronic pain for years after a neck injury from a 1987 car accident. Managing the pain mainly with "Advil and ice packs," she focused her energy not on her career, but on becoming a wife and a mom -- eventually marrying actor Clark Gregg and having daughter Stella, now 9.

When she joined Dancing's 11th season, she did it largely because she wanted to push herself after a surgery to insert a plate in her neck (to ease the pain and prevent further damage). This led doctors to discover cancerous tumors on her thyroid. The cancer had not spread, and her thyroid was removed, and no chemotherapy or radiation was needed.

"I wondered what if I took more risks?" she said. She danced without knowing whether she could complete her final dance -- the night before the finale, she ruptured a disc in her lower back. But even her doctor, who supervised her carefully, said: "People are better off moving around than sitting around." Surgery to repair the disc has left her "pain free."

Tobey Maguire

The *Spider Man* star has had back pain and related problems for several years. His condition has sometimes been aggravated by training for and performing stunts for movies.

Maguire has learned to cope with the pain, and he continues to take on challenging roles.

The star of the blockbuster "Spider-Man" trilogy almost did not make it into his Spidey outfit for the second film, because of the on-

and-off back pain he has had for several years.

"I saw the animatics and the story boards of the stunts that I was to do on *Spider-Man 2*, and I was a little concerned about it," Maguire said in an interview with *Sci Fi Weekly*. "I felt it was my responsibility to disclose my back discomfort to the studio, and to the insurance company, and to the filmmakers, which I did. They were understandably concerned."

Maguire said his condition was likely worsened by the horse riding required for his role in the Academy Award-nominated movie "Seabiscuit," during the previous year.

Though Maguire may have felt obliged to disclose pertinent medical information to the filmmakers, many actors may have gone on with the show, even if it meant performing dangerous stunts, rather than losing a plum role because of chronic pain.

Performing their own stunts gives actors credibility with an audience. But ultimately, if they are not properly trained, they may put themselves at greater risk for injury, Chisholm said.

"We want to believe he is actually playing that role, and the actors feel that," he said. "But when you ignore pain and don't try to address it, it leads to long-term chronic disorders."

PART FIVE
NEW PARADIAGM FOR A PAIN-FREE BACK, A STRONG SPINE, AND A VIBRANT LIFE

Medical sciences and arts have made great progresses in the past century. A lot of suffering has been prevented and eliminated. Unfortunately, the artificial world around us has also been evolving further against the evolution of our spine and back. As a result, back pain has become increasingly prevalent. The approaches we have adopted in dealing with our back and spinal health in the past is not capable of dealing with today's challenges. A new paradigm has become urgently necessary.

1

New Paradigm

We know the old status quo is not working. From the dominant understanding and perceptions about spinal health, to the literature and advice available to people suffering from spinal or back problems and those wishing to prevent them, to the way in which various spinal and back healthcare disciplines are integrated or fragmented, and to out dated national policies strategies and systems

A new paradigm is urgently needed. But what should this new paradigm be, to be able to meet the challenges of the new age? No one has the silver-bullet answer. However, based on our discussion in the previous chapters, the following must be the cornerstones of this new paradigm.

1. Realize the Vulnerability of Your Spine

Many back pain sufferers have been told that the spine is one of the strongest parts of our body. However, the staggering statistics that 30 percent of adult Americans are afflicted by back pain each year indicates the contrary. The fact that the spine doesn't easily fall apart doesn't mean that it is not vulnerable.

Most back pains and injuries are the result of repetitive strains. The fact that you are not presently experiencing pain in your back does not mean that your back is not already suffering micro injuries, whether they are in your spinal discs, vertebrae, or your back muscles, tendons, or ligaments. The first time you experience pain in your back is, in most cases, due to the last bit of incremental pressure, load, wear or tear. What breaks a camel's back is the last straw on its back. The author has come across countless back pain patients who personally told me that their back pain (often caused by herniated discs) erupted in their back one day when they were standing or sitting without doing anything special and without anything special happening to them. These are clear cases where the patients' spinal discs had suffered accumulative damages long before they finally gave up, began to interfere with the spinal nerves, and caused the pain in the back.

In fact, in most adults are already suffering various degrees of micro injuries in their spines and the muscles tendons and ligaments around them, especially in the case of people who often sit for prolong periods whether at home, at work or on the road, in the case of people who often have to bend their back forward whether in factories, garden, or at construction sites, and in the case of people who often needs to lift heavy weights whether for work or for sport. If your back and spine are continuously taken for granted, the pain emerging in your back is just a matter of time.

Without realizing how vulnerable our spines are, the appropriate care and maintenance that our back and spine deserve and need, become an illusion, and unnecessary injury and pain become a logical outcome.

The first thing to do towards a healthy back is to stop thinking your spine is one of the strongest parts of your body. Stop abusing it. And start taking care of it immediately. If anyone tries to convince you otherwise, ask them why back pain happens to 80% of people and is becoming more and more prevalent, and point out to them that the fact that they are not presently experiencing back pain does not mean their backs are not already injured. By further taking their back and spine for granted, pain in erupt in their back one day, and the last straw is certainly going to break the camel's back.

2. Realize the Importance of Your Spine

A healthy spine doesn't just mean that you are pain free. In fact, your life is on top of it. From your freedom, to your sexuality, to your vitality, to your youth, to your financial wellbeing, to your relationship, to your productivity, to your happiness, everything is at stake.

Give your spine more credit that is long overdue. Appreciate your spine more. Learn more about it. Do more for it. Be more careful when using it.

3. Take Care of Your Spine as You Do with Your Teeth

Unfortunately, despite such critical importance, most people take far more care of their teeth and face, than of their back and spine.

Take more care of it. Invest more to protect it. Exercise more to strengthen it. Give at least the same, if not doubled the amount of attention, effort, and resources for your spine and back as for your teeth and face.

Use them properly. Give them the support they need. Give them the protection they need. Give them the exercises they need. Give them the care they need when in pain or discomfort.

4. Realize the Limitations of Your Doctors

As discussed before, there are at least three categories for the origins for back pain. Each of these categories is handled by more than one specialized healthcare discipline that demands lifelong learning, training, and practicing. No one discipline has all the answers.

Also realize that not all doctors and therapists are the same, just like the different shades of a color, such as gray. Some healthcare professionals pass their professional qualification exams with full marks. Others pass them barely with the minimum required points.

You must take responsibility to find the right caregiver, for the right care for your particular situation.

5. Become a Partner with Your Doctor

Doctors are busy. Even if your doctor is the best guru in the world, he or she may not have all the time in the world for your diagnosis and treatment. You must become a partner to your doctor, in your own diagnosis and treatment.

You must provide the right information and ask the right questions to help your own diagnosis. You must actively provide your own experiences and thoughts on your own treatment. You must resist any invasive treatment before you exhaust all other options with other disciplines of care.

6. Clinicians Need to Actively Collaborate for Multidisciplinary Care

In the past century, not only have conventional medical sciences made great progress in back and spinal health but many other disciplines of healthcare have also made great progress. There is a new balance of competence among the various healthcare practitioners for back and spine health.

Clinicians must realize the limitations of their own discipline of care, and appreciate the strength of other disciplines of care for back and spinal health diagnosis and treatment. They must actively seek opinions from their colleagues from other disciplines of care in diagnosing and treating back pain sufferers.

Evidence-based medicine doesn't necessarily mean passing the proof of double blind conventional medicine studies. Otherwise, some effective treatment options for back pain, such as acupuncture, could not have helped countless patients relieve their suffering. What can't be proven, according to the conventional, clinical study standards, may be an indication of the limitation of today's science and technology, instead of that of a particular discipline or method of care. As long as the empirical evidences support the effectiveness of that care, it should be given the credit and consideration that it is due.

7. Don't Take NO for an Answer

"NO" is often the indication of the limitation of a given caregiver or of a given discipline or method of care. Due to the complexity of back and spinal issues, no one care giver or discipline of care could ever have all the answers.

Go and see other caregivers or other disciplines or methods of care for solutions, if someone tells you that the cause of your back pain can't be identified, or your pain can't be relieved, without silencing the alarm systems of your body. You should only allow your body's alarm system to be silenced if you clearly know what the cause is and silencing the alarm system will not interfere with the successful treatment of the cause.

Don't let anyone tell you that you have to live with your pain for the rest of your life. Keep searching. There is a solution for you out there.

8. Adopt New Healthy Lifestyles and Habits

We all know that the right habits and lifestyle are critical. What most people may not appreciate enough is the fact that sitting is the new smoking. Sitting is a leading cause for the occurrence, exaggeration and repetition of back injuries and pain.

The culprit of sitting for back injuries and pains is physical inactivity in the back, along with slouching. You must breakdown the physical inactivity while sitting. Traditional static ergonomics can't help. Find ways to keep the motion in your back even while sitting.

9. Be Your Own First Line of Defense

No one could possibly know you, as well as you do. To find the right care and caregiver for your particular situation, you must take active responsibilities for yourself. You must learn and make an effort to assure you have the right care, right caregiver, right diagnosis and right treatment. Review the previous chapters on how to do it right.

10. Empower integration and prevention in the healthcare policies, strategies, and systems

Non-conventional, non-drug and non-surgery-based care plays a far more important role in spine and back healthcare than in most other areas of healthcare for the management of such diseases such as cold, flu, cardio vascular problems, and cancer.

"Alternative" medicine is no longer alternative in spine and back healthcare. In many, if not most, cases, they are often the most effective cares. They deserve and ought to be among the primary cares in the fight against spine and back problems and suffering. They must be given more credit and consideration in healthcare policies, strategies, and systems.

Prevention must also be given a higher priority in spinal health management policies, strategies and systems. If we could do a better job in preventing spinal problems, a large number of the costly and invasive procedures would become less critical.

One ounce of prevention is worth a pound of cure for patients. In our national healthcare system, one ounce of prevention would be worth a pound of system expenditure and taxpayer money.

By promoting better prevention and devoting five percent of current spinal healthcare costs on prevention, the related national expenditure could be reduced by 30 percent. Such great cost reduction doesn't only mean a savings of $60 to – $80 billion dollars in direct the costs of treating back pain and taxpayers' money, but also a savings of the 70 million otherwise lost work days and productivities in the economy, each year, in the US alone.

JOIN THE MOVEMENT

Join me to call Da Vinci's David out. Together we can call David out earlier and faster. The earlier we can do it, the earlier the millions of back pain sufferers will begin to benefit.

Please email me at *Author@MadBackHappyBack.com* with any feedback, thoughts, critiques, corrections, and suggestions. I shall make my best effort to have your input incorporated in the next edition of this book. Should incorporating your input demand expertise beyond the boundary of my own, I shall have the appropriate experts involved meet the challenge. As soon as your input is incorporated in this book, no matter how small, you will be acknowledged in this book, and will receive a free copy of the next edition.

To help improve this book, you don't necessarily need to be a doctor or any other kind of expert. Often opinions from people who are not experts prove to be the most helpful.

Back and spine health and healing is a complex topic. No one healthcare discipline, let alone any single professional, has all the answers. However, together, we can call David out of the stone. Together, we can help the millions of sufferers stop the hurting. Together, we can help the world cut back pain by at least half.

Let's let the movement begin. Contact me, today!

APPENDIX 1
SPINE ANATOMY

Vertebra

The human spine has a total of 33 vertebrae. Twenty-four of them are separated by spinal discs and are mainly responsible for the unique human functional capability of an upright body position. The other nine vertebrae are not separated and play an assistive role in supporting the human body in an upright position. Five of these nine vertebrae are fused in the pelvis to form the sacrum, and four are fused together to form the tail.

The front part of the vertebrae is large and, depending on its location in the spine, may have a significant wedge shape. This large front part is responsible for taking the total load of the body, above the level of the vertebrae.

The back part of the vertebra is small, intricate with canals to protect the spinal cord and the nerves and provides exits at both left and right sides of this structure for the nerves to branch out of the spinal cord to cover the body.

The spinal cord is the most important part of the spine and the central conductor or source of all pain. It is a long bundle of nervous tissue, extending from the brain to the space between the first and second lumbar vertebrae. The remainder of the spinal canal contains only the branch nerves from the cord.

The fact that the spinal cord stops above the lumbar spine is another evidence of the intelligence and marvel of our body, because the lumbar spine has to take on the countless twisting and bending, which makes it significantly less capable of protecting the spinal cord had the cord extended into this part of the spine. You may say the neck is equally vulnerable as is the lumbar spine. Unfortunately, the neck is the necessary bottle neck, if the spinal cord is to reach into our body. Otherwise, the spinal cord would have stopped in our head.

The brain and the spinal cord together make up the central nervous system. Protecting the spinal cord is as critical as protecting the brain.

Along the entire spine from the neck to the lower back, including the sacrum, nerves branch out from the spinal cord through the spaces between the vertebrae. These out branching nerves spread out over our entire body to control all conscious and subconscious functions of each and every one of our body parts and organs.

Thanks to these nerves, we are able to walk and dance. Thanks to these nerves, we are able to read and write. Thanks to these nerves, we are able to breath and digest. These nerves are critical to all functions of our body. Any nerve injured, damaged or interfered with will not only lead to aches and pains in the back and related body parts, but also lead to malfunction of related body parts or organs. Failing to understand this fact causes countless unnecessary suffering.

The intricate structure is also responsible for coordinating the motions of the adjacent vertebra and to set a proper range of bending and twisting motions for the spine. This intricate structure at the back of the vertebra also sets special space for a sophisticated network of stabilizing muscles and ligaments to attach to and to hold the spinal vertebrae together and aligned. While the ligaments house and hold the spine together, the muscles stabilize the spine, and control its motion.

Discs

Between the vertebral bones are intervertebral discs. The discs have a gel-like core (nucleus) that shifts, buffers, and distributes spinal pressure. Encasing the gel-like core are two layers of exceedingly tough, strong yet flexible shells, the inner annulus and outer annulus. The annulus are so strong that the disc is stronger than vertebral body in taking compression forces, which is one of the reasons that compression fractures of the vertebral body could happen.

While the inner annulus mainly serves as an incasing mechanism to the nucleus, the outer annulus also serves as a protective mechanism because it is filled with pain sensing nerves (sinuvertebral nerves). By sending pain signals, the sinuvertebral nerves tells the brain that the pressure on the spine is too high or the spinal disc is damaged or about to be damaged that the body needs to react quickly to avoid further consequences.

Since aging weakens the discs, the pain sensing nerves grow in density to make sure to be able to send out pain signals when needed. The fact that you may experience more pain is an indication of your body's natural ingenuity in self-protection. The separation by spinal discs gives the vertebrae the ability to accommodate the movement of the spine. The spinal discs allow the spine to bend forward, backward, and sideways, and allows the spine to twist and the body to rotate.

Besides the obvious purpose of such bending and twisting, this function is critical to allow the body to shift its weight to make walking possible. It also absorbs shocks to the human brain, and allows the distribution of the central nerves to various parts of our body by creating perfect passages between the vertebrae for the nerve branches. Without spinal discs, the central nerves either can't be effectively distributed to our extremities and organs, or can't be properly protected in our body against environmental impact. Spinal discs are a critical part of the spine and contributes to a quarter of its length.

Constantly in motion and supporting most of the body weight and external weight load our body carries, it takes on most of the wear and tear of the spine. Healthy discs automatically act to evenly distribute the weight and pressure throughout the entire disc area. However, this capability decreases as the discs get worn, torn and become more and more degenerated. This is one of the reasons why you need to pay more and more attention to your spine when you age.

The perfect shape and construction of the 24 disc-separated vertebrae not only allows the bending, twisting, and turning, but also allows the perfect balance of our body. These 24 flexible vertebrae are separated into three sections of our spine for distinct functions. Although during the embryogenesis (early stage of pregnancy), all vertebrae are aligned in one big C curve, within the first year or two these 24 vertebrae will gradually form themselves into three distinct spinal curves - the lower back curve (lumbar lordotic curve), upper back curve (thoracic kyphotic curve), and the neck curve (cervical lordotic curve).

Lower back (lumbar spine) — Most of us have five vertebrae numbered L1 to L5 (from top to bottom) in our lumbar spine. The lumbar spine, which connects the thoracic spine and the pelvis, bears the bulk of the body's weight – the lower in the lumbar spine, the higher the load on a given lumbar vertebrae, and the thicker or larger the lumbar vertebrae itself, with L5 being the largest one. L1 to L5 form our lumbar curve which concaves backwards.

Upper back (thoracic spine) — our upper back spine consists of 12 vertebrae (T1 to T12 from top to bottom). The ribs attach to the spine on the thoracic vertebrae, which form the forward concaving thoracic curve of our spine – the second curve from the top of our spine. Why is this curve opposite to the first curve? We will discuss it later.

Neck (cervical spine) — our neck is the uppermost section of our spine. Our neck consists of seven vertebrae, numbered C1 to C7 from top to bottom. These seven vertebrae form the uppermost curve of our spine. This curve concaves backward and performs vital functions to our body. The first two vertebrae of the cervical spine are specialized to allow for head movement. C1 (also called the atlas, which is named after the primordial Titan Atlas, in Greek mythology, who holds the world on his back,) sits between the skull and the rest of the spine. C2 (also called the axis) has a projection that fits within a hole in the atlas (C1) to allow rotation of the head.

Spinal curves are essential to protect the human brain from shocks coming up from walking and running, because the brain is directly on the top of the spine. If the spine is straight, any shock from the ground will be directly transmitted to the brain. The spinal curvature is a further shock absorbing and diffusing mechanism of the spine, in addition to the spinal discs. The perfect arrangement of the various curves along the spine is essential to allow our head to be in an upright position.

The backward concaving lower back curve provides our body with maximum ability to lift heavy objects such as our children, our drinking water, harvest our crops, use building materials -- the essential activities to human survival. However, with only a backward concaving lower back curve, the human body would not be able to main a sustainable upright posture. To combat this dilemma, nature created a counter balancing forward concaving upper back curve which balances the gravity centers of the lower body and upper body on the center line when we stand up.

However, if a human head is aligned with the forward concaving upper back curve, we would forever only be able to face our feet instead of looking forward. The backwards concaving neck curve came to the rescue. Our neck curvature is therefore the key for humans to be able to hold the head up right.

By now, do you not wonder how our spine has been developed so perfectly? Don't you think our spine is a true piece of wonder?

By understanding the remarkable design and function of our spine, you would also understand the importance of the curves. Maintaining a healthy curvature in all the above discussed spinal curves is absolutely essential for the proper function of our body.

Despite the wonderful shape and construction of our spine, it is one of the most sensitive parts of our body. Malfunction of the spine often brings serious even devastating consequences to our health, productivity, life quality, freedom, and happiness.

The most sensitive parts of the spine are the lower back and the neck. That is why debilitating lower back pain and nagging neck pain are so pervasive.

Ligaments

Ligaments around the spine facilitate the motion of the spine from flexion, extension, and rotation. There are a number of ligaments in the intricate ligament system protecting the spine and spinal cord, while allowing spinal motion. The range of motion of each vertebra is limited by its associated ligaments and muscles as well as the shape of the vertebra. Despite these limitations, the combined range of motion of many or all vertebrae is significant and makes our bending, twisting, and daily activity a reality.

Anterior longitudinal ligament is a broad band of ligaments consisting of three layers of ligaments going from C1 to sacrum. The most superficial layer of the ligaments extends over four to five vertebrae, the middle layer of ligaments extends over two to three vertebrae, and the inner most layer extends from one vertebra to the next.

The posterior longitudinal ligament is inside the vertebral canal forward attached to the main column of the spine vertebrae. It also extends the entire spine, and plays a major role in keeping the vertebrae in place, like a kebab skewer holding pieces of food together. Injury to the posterior longitudinal ligament is common in improper lifting activities. Weakened or torn posterior longitudinal ligaments often leads to herniated, or slipped discs. (Slouching while sitting is one of the leading ways to weaken posterior longitudinal ligaments.)

The supraspinous ligament is a thick cord of ligament connecting the outer most tips of vertebrae from C7 to sacrum. The interspinous ligament is the intermittent ligament tissue that connects adjacent vertebrae through the length of the backward protruding bone spikes (spinous process). Intertransverse ligaments connect adjacent vertebrae along the length of the sideways protruding bony wings (transverse process). Intertransverse ligaments are interwoven with the deep back muscles (intertransversarii muscles).

Ligamentum flavum connects the lamina of adjacent vertebrae through the entire spine to the sacrum. It helps maintain an upright posture.

Muscles

There are six layers of muscles in the back. The first and most superficial layer consists of the power muscles trapezius and latissumus dorsi. The second layer consists of levator scapula, rhomboid major, and minor. The third layer consists of serratus posterior superior and inferior. The fourth layer consists of splenius capitis and cervisis. The fifth layer consists of iliocostalis, longissimus, and spinalis. The sixth and inner most layer consists of semispinalis, multifidis, rotators, interspinalis, intertransverarii, and levator costarum.

The deeper the layer, the finer and shorter the muscles, and the more difficult to exercise and strengthen. Most back pain involves multifidis, rotators, interspinalis, and intertransverarii, because they are directly responsible for the fine control of the bending and twisting movement of the spine, and most people have a relative weakness in these muscles. The superficial power muscles remain in good condition without injury in most cases of back pain.

Pelvis

If the spine is the foundation of the back, then the pelvis is the foundation of the spine. It is the foundation of the foundation. Its optimal form and function are the determining factors for the health of your spine, hence your back. Of course, while you are on your legs, your legs and feet are in turn the foundation of your pelvis, hence your spine and back. That is the reason why the origins of many back pains are in the feet or legs.

APPENDIX II
SURGERIES AND DRUGS FOR
BACK PAIN MANAGEMENT

Surgery

In chronic back pain relief, surgery operates on two main promises.

1. Decompress a nerve root that is pinched, and
2. Stabilize a painful joint, according to Dr. Peter Ullrich a spine surgeon in Appleton, Wisconsin.

Surgery must be considered as the last option, because besides its high side effects and high costs, its success predictability is uncertain except for a limited range of conditions, such as discectomy (or microdiscectomy) for a lumbar disc herniation that is causing leg pain or a spine fusion for spinal instability.

Surgery's uncertainty is so high that there exists a term "Failed Back Surgery Syndrome" (FBSS) or Failed Back Syndrome (FBS) or Post-Laminectomy Syndrome (PLS) to describe a condition characterized by persistent pain following back surgeries.

There are many reasons for a back surgery to end up in FBSS. For example, the fusion of vertebrae may fail, or the metal implant for the fusion may fail. Also a fusion may lead to acceleration of degeneration in adjacent spinal disc and or vertebrae, the lesion may transfer to such affected vertebrae or discs. Decompression of a nerve root may be inadequate. Preoperative nerve damage may not heal after a decompressive surgery. Unexpected nerve damage may occur during a surgery. A nonphysiologic scar on the nerve (epidural fibrosis) may form which, from the very onset, behaves as a reparative inflammation causing clinical problems and pain. Damage of the soft tissue may lead to pain. After recovery the connective tissue may create fybrosis that traps the pain receptors. Hence, myofascial pain may happen post-surgery.

Post-surgery back pain may also continue due to other reasons. Studies have found that cigarette smokers suffer greater risk with failed spinal surgery that aim to decrease back pain and spinal impairment. Nicotine has been found to interfere with bone metabolism and restrict small blood vessel diameter leading to increased scar formation post operation. In a year-long study in 1987, researchers found that smoking history (current and ex-smokers) dramatically increased the risk for both herniated disc in lower back (prolapsed lumbar intervertebral disc) (56 percent versus 37 percent of controls) and disc diseases in the neck (cervical disc disease) (64.3 percent versus 37 percent of controls).

The study ran from 1987-1988, and had 205 cigarette smoking surgical patients with back pain (163 patients with lumbar disc disease and 42 patients with cervical disc disease) and compared these smokers to 205 age-sex-matched non-smoking inpatient controls. The study was conducted at the Pennsylvania Hospital in Philadelphia, Pennsylvania.

Surgery can't treat all pain generators. It is not a ultimate once-for-all treatment for all back pains. In fact, it is NOT even an effective choice for most back pains, even if it does not have any side effects or potential risks that are inherent with it.

Surgery may significantly alter the biomechanics of the spine. For example, in the case of spinal fusion in the lower back, two or more vertebrae are fused together and function as one unit. This leads to a reduction in the number of vertebrae and discs that can facilitate the bending and twisting of the spine, which increases the stress on adjacent vertebrae and discs. This not only reduces the range of motion of the patient but also increases the wear, tear, inflammation, and degeneration of the adjacent spine, due to overuse, which may cause the pain lesion to migrate to these adjacent spinal blocks, which is referred to as Adjacent Segment Disease.

Before considering surgery, it is helpful for patients to research and be informed about Adjacent Segment Disease and its related discussions online and in literature.

Drugs

There are many categories of drugs. No matter what category of drug you are attempting to take, take it with caution.

All drugs have side effects, especially if you take them at higher doses for a prolonged period. For example, Tylenol is the number one cause of acute liver failure in the States. Acute liver failure related to the use of the acetaminophen-based painkiller rose from 28 percent of all cases in 1998, to 51 percent in 2003. Tylenol, along with other acetaminophen-containing combination drugs, kills hundreds of people and send about 56,000 more to the hospital each year in the States alone. (for further details, google "Tylenol liver damage.")

Most pain killers lead to constipation. All Nonsteroidal anti-inflammatory drugs (NSAIDs) can cause stomach irritation. Often patients are forced to take secondary drugs to treat the side effects of the primary medicine. And the secondary drugs also have their own side effects, which people either have to deal with or have to take a third drug to treat… and on and on the cycle goes.

You should always take the smallest dose required. And you should only take it for as long as you absolutely need it.

In today's society, we have a tendency to over use drugs. Think twice before spending your hard earned cash on those little bottles.

Pain Killers

One of the first things that back pain sufferers take for back pain are pain killers. Most pain killers are acetaminophen-based such as

- Actamin,
- Panadol,
- Tylenol, (most prominent and well-known)
- Anacin,
- Excedrin.

Despite the many brands, all pain killers work the same way. They stop or cut off the transmission of pain signals from the pain receptors to the brain. It is like your home alarm system. When a burglar enters your home, your home alarm system will send loud and annoying warnings to you and you feel really disturbed, distracted, and upset.

To avoid such distractions, you have several options. First, you can strengthen your home so that no burglar can enter. Second, you may find a guard to subdue the burglar as soon as he enters your home. Third, you may choose to cut the wires connecting the sensors and the alarm so the alarm will not sound, but the burglar is still in your home.

Pain killers work like the third option above. It doesn't mean that your pain or its cause is no longer there when you use pain killers. It only means that you don't feel the pain. The pain killer has just numbed you to the sensing of the pain. In a way, the pain killer is fooling your brain by withholding vital warning signals on your health.

In many cases, especially with young people, this can be dangerous. Young people know no limits. As soon as their sense of pain subsides, they tend to think that their body is ok and ready for abuse again. The subsequent careless physical activities may worsen and deepen the original problem, that never went away in the first place. And in terms of recovery, if you continue to burden injured tissues while taking pain killers to numb your senses, you will almost certainly prolong recovery time and possibly cause long-term damage.

Of course, this is not to discredit pain killers. They have their benefits, purposes, and value. Only one must exercise caution when using them. One should only use pain killers:

- If one can't find a timely solution to resolve the cause or the root problem of the pain,
- Or if one needs relief, while in a process of treating the cause or the root problem,
- Or if one has simply run out of possibilities to address the cause of the root problem,
- Or if the pain is phantom pain, which is simply a malfunction of one's own pain sensory system.

Anti-inflammatory Medicine

Only a small portion of back pain is caused by inflammations.

Anti-inflammatory drugs help relieve back pain by suppressing inflammation or inflammation-originated pain causing chemicals in our body. For example, Ibuprofen, one of the most popular anti-inflammatory active ingredients, works by blocking the effects of cyclo-oxygenase (COX) enzymes and reducing the prostaglandins.

Prostaglandins are chemicals produced at sites of injury or damage, in the body and cause pain and inflammation. Blocking the effects of COX enzymes means fewer prostaglandins are produced, which in turn, means less pain and inflammation.

Hence, it becomes clear that anti-inflammatory drugs would only work for you if your back pain is caused by some actual damage in your back tissues. However, a great amount of back pain is not caused by any physical damage and is not associated with any inflammation, such as back pain due to nerve interference or sciatica, in which cases, NSAIDs (nonsteroidal anti-inflammatory drugs) will not be of any help.

Below are the popular Over The Counter (OTC) Non-Steroidal Anti-inflammatory drugs (NSAIDs) for back pain -- listed from the mildest (top of the list), to the strongest (bottom of the list) with associated brands.

- Aspirin - Anacin, Bayer, Bufferin, Ecotrin
- Combination of aspirin and acetaminophen - Vanquish
- Ibuprofen - Advil, Motrin, Nuprin, Medipren
- Naproxen sodium - Aleve, Naproxen
- Ketoprofen - Actron, Orudis

Muscle Relaxants
It is natural for our body, that upon injury, the surrounding muscles start to contract and tend to restrict the motion of the injured area. This process is designed by nature to protect the injured area and to prevent further damage to the area. However, this process also often causes the pain receptors in these muscles to fire and to send pain signals to our brain. As a result, we are not only feeling the pain from the injured area, but also from its surrounding muscles that contract and tense in an attempt to protect us. Thus, your health care giver may also recommend muscle relaxants to you. Here are some of the common muscle relaxants:

- Cyclobenzaprine (Flexeril)
- Tizanidine (Zanaflex)
- Baclofen (Lioresal)
- Carisoprodol (Soma)

Again, these medicines do not help with the root cause of the pain. While the corresponding muscles are forced to relax by the muscle relaxant, the pain of the injured area and the root cause of the pain continue.

Most drugs have uses according to the label and best uses according to Consumer's Guide. The labeled uses may not be the same as the "best uses." Labeled uses are approved by the American Food and Drug Administration (FDA). Best uses are according to consumer experiences and opinions, and may not be completely accurate, but may yield some interesting clues for your decision of which drug may be more suitable to you.

If the effective chemical ingredient(s) is or are the same, chances are that the effect on you will be similar, if not the same. Most differences between different brands or manufacturers would mainly be in the formulation of the inactive supportive substances -- the fillers (excipient) or diluents. In most tablets or injection liquids, up to 99 percent of the total volume or weight may be fillers. These fillers, although not active, have important functions. In most cases, they are formulated to give you the best release of the active ingredients over a period of time, and to allow the best absorption of the active ingredients, or to minimize or prevent irritation or damage to your stomach or digestive tracks. Unfortunately, data or information is rare about the quality of the fillers of each drug. Even if it is available, it could most likely be interpreted only by trained specialists.

REFERENCES

Nachemson AL. Newest knowledge of lower back pain. A critical look. Clin Orthop 1992; Jun: 8–20.

Research on lower back pain and common spinal disorders. NIH GUIDE, Volume 26, Number 16, May 16, 1997, National Institutes of Health. Available from: http://grants2.nih.gov/grants/guide/pa-files/PA-97-058.html

José García-Cosamalón, Miguel E del Valle, Marta G Calavia,Olivia García-Suárez, Alfonso López-Muñiz, Jesús Otero, and José A Vega, "Intervertebral disc, sensory nerves and neurotrophins: who is who in discogenic pain?" Journal of Anatomy, 2010 July; 217(1): 1–15

Neil Osterweil, Robert Jasmer, "Acetaminophen Is Leading Cause of Acute Liver Failure" MedPage Today, Nov 30, 2005

Shereen Jegtvig, "Eating cues thrown off in people with back pain: study", Reuter Health, NEW YORK, Jan 15, 2014, www.reuters.com/article/2014/01/15/us-eating-pain-idUSBREA0E1A220140115

Darrin Pordash, Kari Riemann, Top Ten Chiropractic Techniques, Logan University, Dec. 1997

William J. Lauretti, What are the Risk of Chiropractic Neck Treatments? The American Chiropractic Association, 1996

Dvorak J, Orelli F. How dangerous is manipulation to the cervical spine? Manual Medicine 1985; 2: 1-4.

Jaskoviak P. Complications arising from manipulation of the cervical spine. J Manip Physiol Ther 1980; 3: 213-19.

Henderson DJ, Cassidy JD. Vertebral Artery syndrome. In: Vernon H. Upper cervical syndrome: chiropractic diagnosis and treatment. Baltimore: Williams and Wilkins, 1988: 195-222.

Terrett AG. Vascular accidents from cervical spine manipulation: Report of 107 cases. J Aust Chiro Assoc 1987; 17: 15-24.

Terrett AG, Kleynhans AM. Cerebrovascular complications of manipulation. In: Haldeman S., ed. Principals and Practice of Chiropractic. Norwalk, Ct.: Appleton & Lang, 1992: 579-98.

Jyrki Salmenkivi, Deaths due to medical error during spinal surgery are rare, Spinal News International, Oct 4, 2013

The case for personalized medicine, Personalized medicine coalition, 3rd edition

Grzanna R, Lindmark L, Frondoza CG. Ginger--an herbal medicinal product with broad anti-inflammatory actions. Journal of Medicinal Food. 2005 Summer; 8(2): 125-32.

Zi-Feng Zhanga, Shao-Hua Fana, Yuan-Lin Zhenga, Jun Lua, Dong-Mei Wua, Qun Shana, Bin Hua, Purple sweet potato color attenuates oxidative stress and inflammatory response induced by d-galactose in mouse liver, Food and Chemical Toxicology, Volume 47, Issue 2, February 2009, Pages 496–501

Sleigh, AE, Kuehl KS, Elliot DL . Efficacy of tart cherry juice to reduce inflammation among patients with osteoarthritis. American College of Sports Medicine Annual Meeting. May 30, 2012.

Kuehl KS, Perrier ET, Elliot DL, Chestnutt J. Efficacy of tart cherry juice in reducing muscle pain during running: a randomized controlled trial. Journal of the International Society of Sports Nutrition, 2010; 7:17-22.

Daniel C. Cherkin, Karen J. Sherman, Andrew L. Avins, Janet H. Erro, Laura Ichikawa, William E. Barlow, Kristin Delaney, Rene Hawkes, Luisa Hamilton, Alice Pressman, Partap S. Khalsa, and Richard A. Deyo, A Randomized Trial Comparing Acupuncture, Simulated Acupuncture, and Usual Care for Chronic Lower back Pain, Archive of Internal Medicine. 2009 May 11; 169(9): 858–866, www.ncbi.nlm.nih.gov/pmc/articles/PMC2832641/

Margaret A. Nasser, Neurological Rehabilitation: Acupuncture and Laser Acupuncture To Treat Paralysis in Stroke and Other Paralytic Conditions and Pain in Carpal Tunnel Syndrome, Boston University

Burton AK, Tillotson KM, Main CJ, Hollis S. "Psychosocial predictors of outcome in acute and subchronic lower back trouble". Spine 1995, 20 (6): 722–8.

Dionne CE. "Psychological distress confirmed as predictor of long-term back-related functional limitations in primary care settings". Journal of Clinical Epidemiology, July 2005, Volume 58, Issue 7 , Pages 714-718,

An HS, Silveri CP, Simpson JM, File P, Simmons C, Simeone FA, Balderston RA. Comparison of smoking habits between patients with surgically confirmed herniated lumbar and cervical disc disease and controls, Journal Spinal Disorder. 1994 Oct;7(5):369-73.

Iwahashi, Masaki MD; Matsuzaki, Hiromi MD; Tokuhashi, Yasuaki MD; Wakabayashi, Ken MD; Uematsu, Yoshinao MD, Mechanism of Intervertebral Disc Degeneration Caused by Nicotine in Rabbits to Explicate Intervertebral Disc Disorders Caused by Smoking, Spine, 1 July 2002 - Volume 27 - Issue 13 - pp 1396-1401

Foreman, Stephen M.; Croft, Arthur C. (2002). Whiplash injuries : the cervical acceleration/deceleration syndrom. Philadelphia: Lippincott Williams Wilkins. ISBN 0-7817-2681-6.

Brent Bauer, MD, Mayo Clinic Wellness Solution for Back Pain, Gaiam, 2007

Ellis F. Friedman, MD, Outwitting Back Pain, The Lyons Press, 2004

John E. Sarno, MD, Healing Back Pain, Hachette Book Group, 2010

Webb R, Brammah T, Lunt M, et al. Prevenlence and predictors of intense, chronic, and disabling neck and back pain in the UK general population. Spine 2003; 28: 1195-202

Tim John Sloan, Rajiva Gupta, Weiya Zhang, David Andrew Walsh, Beliefs about the causes and consequences of pain in patients with chronic inflammatory or noninflammatory lower back pain and in pain free individuals. Spine 2008; 33 (9): 966-972

Stewart WF, et al. Lost productive time and cost due to common pain conditions in the US workforce. JAMA. 2003 Nov 12; 290 (18): 2443-54

H.R Guo, S Tanaka, W E Halperin, L L Cameron, Back pain prevalence in US industry and estimates of lost work days, American Journal of Public Health, 1999, July; 89(7): 1029-35

Relief for your aching back - What worked for our readers, The Consumer Reports Health Ratings Center, March 2013

Dr. Michael Peters, Dr. John Tanner, Eva Niezgoda-Hadjidemetri, Essential Back Care, DK Publishing, 2011

Keefe, F. J. (2011). Behavioral medicine: a voyage to the future. Annals of Behavioral Medicine, 41, 141-151

John E. Sarno, MD, Healing Back Pain: The Mind-Body Connection, Reed Business Information, Inc. 1999

Notarnicola A1, Fischetti F, Maccagnano G, Comes R, Tafuri S, Moretti B. Daily pilates exercise or inactivity for patients with lower back pain: a clinical prospective observational study. European Journal of Physical and Rehabilitation Medicine. 2014 Feb; 50(1):59-66.

Paul Little, et al. Randomised controlled trial of Alexander technique lessons, exercise, and massage (ATEAM) for chronic and recurrent back pain. BMJ, 337, August 19, 2008; www.bmj.com/content/337/bmj.a884

Woodman JP1, Moore NR. Evidence for the effectiveness of Alexander Technique lessons in medical and health-related conditions: a systematic review. International Journal of Clinical Practice. 2012 Jan;66(1):98-112. doi: 10.1111/j.1742-1241.2011.02817.x.

Connors KA1, Pile C, Nichols ME. Does the Feldenkrais Method make a difference? An investigation into the use of outcome measurement tools for evaluating changes in clients. Journal Bodywork Movement Therapies. 2011 Oct;15(4):446-52. doi: 10.1016/j.jbmt.2010.09.001.

Lake, Bernard (1992). Photoanalysis of Standing Posture in Controls and Lower back Pain: Effects of Kinesthetic Processing (Feldenkrais Method sessions) in Posture and Gait: Control Mechanisms VII. eds. M Woollocott and F Horak, U of Oregon Press, , pp 400- 403.

Peng PW. Tai chi and chronic pain. Regional Anesthesia and Pain Medicine, 2012 Jul-Aug; 37(4):372-82. doi: 10.1097/AAP.0b013e31824f6629.

Hall AM1, Maher CG, Lam P, Ferreira M, Latimer J. Tai chi exercise for treatment of pain and disability in people with persistent lower back pain: a randomized controlled trial. Arthritis Care & Research (Hoboken). 2011 Nov;63(11):1576-83. doi: 10.1002/acr.20594.

Cramer H1, Lauche R, Haller H, Dobos G. A systematic review and meta-analysis of yoga for lower back pain. The Clinical Journal of Pain. 2013 May;29(5):450-60. doi: 10.1097/AJP.0b013e31825e1492.

Robert B. Saper, 1 ,* Ama R. Boah, 1 Julia Keosaian, 1 Christian Cerrada, 1 Janice Weinberg, 2 and Karen J. Sherman. Comparing Once- versus Twice-Weekly Yoga Classes for Chronic Lower back Pain in Predominantly Low Income Minorities: A Randomized Dosing Trial. Evidence Based Complement Alternative Medicine. 2013; 2013: 658030.

Nikoobakht, Fraidouni, Yaghoubidoust, Burri, Pakpour. Sexual function and associated factors in Iranian patients with chronic lower back pain. Spinal Cord. 2014 Apr;52(4):307-12. doi: 10.1038/sc.2013.151.

Ramsey S. Opioids for back pain are linked to increased risk of erectile dysfunction. BMJ. 2013 May 17;346:f3223. doi: 10.1136/bmj.f3223.

Ferreira PH1, Pinheiro MB, Machado GC, Ferreira ML. Is alcohol intake associated with lower back pain? A systematic review of observational studies. Manual Therapy. 2013 Jun;18(3):183-90. doi: 10.1016/j.math.2012.10.007. Epub 2012 Nov 10.

Ahn NU, Ahn UM, Nallamshetty L, Buchowski JM, Rose PS, Sponseller PD. Lumbar spine pathology and atherosclerotic risk factors: a 53-year prospective study of 1337 patients. TRANS AAOS, 68:155, 2001, The Spine Journal, Volume 2, Issue 2, Supplement 1 , Page 34, March 2002

Jerosch, Jörg; Heisel, Jürgen, Management der Arthrose: Innovative Therapiekonzepte, Deutscher Ärzteverlag. p. 107. ISBN 978-3-7691-0599-5.

Singh, Arun Kumar, The Comprehensive History of Psychology. Motilal Banarsidass Publ. p. 66. ISBN 978-81-208-0804-1.

Dickinson, John, Proprioceptive control of human movement. p. 4. Princeton Book Co., 1976, ISBN 860190021

Foster, Susan Leigh, Choreographing Empathy: Kinesthesia in Performance. Taylor & Francis. p. 74. ISBN 978-0-415-59655-8.

Brookhart, John M.; Mountcastle, Vernon B. Geiger, Stephen R. The Nervous system: Sensory processes ; volume editor: Ian Darian-Smith. American Physiological Society. p. 784. ISBN 978-0-683-01108-1.

Magnusson SP1, Simonsen EB, Aagaard P, Gleim GW, McHugh MP, Kjaer M. Viscoelastic response to repeated static stretching in the human hamstring muscle. Scandinavian Journal of Medicine and Science in Sports. 1995 Dec;5(6):342-7.

Taylor DC1, Dalton JD Jr, Seaber AV, Garrett WE Jr. Viscoelastic properties of muscle-tendon units. The biomechanical effects of stretching. American Journal of Sports Medicine. 1990 May-Jun;18(3):300-9.

Keitaro Kubo, Hiroaki Kanehisa, Yasuo Kawakami, Tetsuo Fukunaga, Influence of static stretching on viscoelastic properties of human tendon structures in vivo, Journal of Applied PhysiologyPublished 1 February 2001Vol. 90no. 520-527

Alan R. Stockard, Thomas Wesley Allen, Competence Levels in Musculoskeletal

Medicine: Comparison of Osteopathic and Allopathic Medical Graduates, Journal of the American Osteopathic Association, www.jaoa.org/content/106/6/350.full.pdf, accessed on July 2nd, 2014

Kristina Åkesson, Karsten E. Dreinhöfer, A.D.Woolf, Improved education in musculoskeletal conditions is necessary for all doctors, Bulletin of the World Health Organization, 2003; 81(9): 677–683.

Oh DY, Talukdar S, Bae EJ, Imamura T, Morinaga H, Fan W, Li P, Lu WJ, Watkins SM, Olefsky JM, GPR120 is an omega-3 fatty acid receptor mediating potent anti-inflammatory and insulin-sensitizing effects, Cell. 2010 Sep 3;142(5):687-98

Dyszkiewicz A, Opara J. Monitoring the treatment of low back pain using non-steroid anti-inflammatory drugs and aromatic oil components, Ortopedia Traumatologia Rehabilitacja, 2006 Apr 28;8(2):210-8.

Sritoomma N, Moyle W, Cooke M, O'Dwyer S, The effectiveness of Swedish massage with aromatic ginger oil in treating chronic low back pain in older adults: a randomized controlled trial, Complementary Therapies in Medicine, 2014 Feb;22(1):26-33. doi: 10.1016/j.ctim.2013.11.002. Epub 2013 Nov 12

Yip YB, Tse SH, The effectiveness of relaxation acupoint stimulation and acupressure with aromatic lavender essential oil for non-specific low back pain in Hong Kong: a randomized controlled trial. Complement Ther Med. 2004 Mar;12(1):28-37.

Bahouq H1, Fadoua A, Hanan R, Ihsane H, Najia HH. Profile of sexuality in Moroccan chronic low back pain patients. BMC Musculoskeletal Disorders, 2013 Feb 15;14:63. doi: 10.1186/1471-2474-14-63.

Douglas M. Gillard, Associate Professor, Palmer College of Chiropractic, Lumbar Spine & Disc Anatomy,
www.chirogeek.com/Anatomy%20Page/disc-anatomy.html
Clayton Scott, Associate Professor, University of Michigan, Repetitive Strain Injury,
http://web.eecs.umich.edu/~cscott/rsi.html

www.ingramcontent.com/pod-product-compliance
Lightning Source LLC
Chambersburg PA
CBHW020657270326
41928CB00005B/163